To Leo —

One good book
deserves another

[signature]

July 62

Behavioral Changes
in Patients
Following Strokes

Publication Number 474

AMERICAN LECTURE SERIES®

A Monograph in

AMERICAN LECTURES IN PHYSICAL MEDICINE
AND REHABILITATION

Edited by

W. A. SELLE, Ph.D., M.D.
*Clinical Professor of Physical Medicine
and Rehabilitation
Professor of Biophysics
University of California Medical School
Los Angeles, California*

By

MONTAGUE ULLMAN, M.D.

Director of Psychiatry
Maimonides Hospital of Brooklyn
Associate Professor of Psychiatry
State University of New York
Downstate Medical Center
Formerly, Psychiatrist, Stroke Study
Bellevue Hospital, New York City

Behavioral Changes
in Patients
Following Strokes

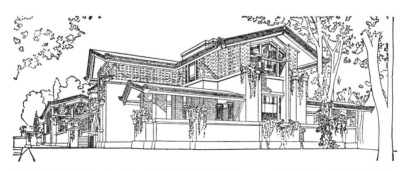

CHARLES C THOMAS · PUBLISHER
Springfield · Illinois · U.S.A.

CHARLES C THOMAS • PUBLISHER

Bannerstone House

301-327 East Lawrence Avenue, Springfield, Illinois, U.S.A.

*With THOMAS BOOKS careful attention is given to all details of
manufacturing and design. It is the Publisher's desire to present books
that are satisfactory as to their physical qualities and artistic possibilities
and appropriate for their particular use. THOMAS BOOKS will be
true to those laws of quality that assure a good name and good will.*

Printed in the United States of America

PREFACE

In July, 1956, a long-range study of cerebrovascular disease was initiated at Bellevue Hospital in New York City. The chief aims were to establish a more accurate knowledge of the natural history of the various syndromes subsumed under the term "cerebrovascular disease" and to evaluate the efficacy of anticoagulant therapy and rehabilitation procedures. The study was supported by a grant from the National Institute of Neurological Diseases and Blindness (U. S. Public Health Service Grant No. 3-B-9009). An unusual opportunity existed in connection with this study for the collection of data on the psychological aspects of patients with strokes in both the acute and chronic phases of their illness. Empirical observations attested to the role of personality in accounting for differing responses of patients during the recovery process. A retrospective study on patients with hemiparesis or hemiplegia due to cerebrovascular disease emphasized motivation as the single most important factor influencing recovery (1). Furthermore, no large-scale psychiatric studies had appeared concerned with the problems of stroke patients, particularly in the early stages of their illness.

Accordingly, in March, 1957, a psychiatric team comprising a psychiatrist, a psychologist and a psychiatric social worker was organized to work in conjunction with the medical, neurological and rehabilitation personnel. The psychiatric data to be presented are based on observations made over a three-year period (1957-1960). The patients selected were admitted to the stroke study at Bellevue Hospital after a diagnosis of cerebrovascular disease had been established. The main categories of strokes included those due to thrombosis, embolism and hemorrhage. A smaller group consisted of those patients with recurrent transient intermittent ischemic episodes. The diagnoses as given in the case presentations were either substantiated by angiographic studies or else represent a generalized site description as established clinically. The patient population fell in the lower socio-economic level and included, in the stroke age group, a majority of patients who were foreign born. Patients were not included in the psychiatric study when systematic observations were not possible either because of the severity of the medical condition or the existence of language barriers. The total number of patients seen during the three-year period was 300.

Throughout the text the term "stroke" is used as it appears to be the most familiar and most meaningful designation applied to the group of cerebrovascular diseases. This term, as it applies to cerebrovascular phenomena, has been defined as "a focal neurologic process in blood vessels. In addition to its focal character the most essential feature is its *temporal profile* which is characterized by abrupt onset and rapid evolution, the symptoms usually reaching a peak of severity in seconds, minutes, or hours; if not at once fatal, a partial or complete recovery usually occurs in a period of hours, days, weeks or months" (2).

The behavioral changes occurring in the wake of a stroke encompass a wide and varied range of responses. A mild stroke may go undetected both by the patient and those about him. The entire experience may be accompanied by a clear sensorium, insight and appropriate affective responses. Quite often, however, certain distortions may be noted and inappropriate emotional responses occur. The initial phase may be characterized by varying degrees of clouding of consciousness with confusion, disorientation and the occurrence of altered forms of symbolic expression. The mental changes involved may clear up rapidly or slowly, may endure with little change or may become progressively worse. Paradoxically, some aspects of the initial responses may improve, whereas others show little or no change. A severe stroke may result in the loss of consciousness, global aphasia and, in some instances, the rapid onset of a moribund state.

The symptomatology of stroke patients thus taps a potentially wide spectrum of possible behavioral manifestations. The intent of this book is to present a sampling of the variety of behavioral responses that do occur. Abstracts from the clinical protocols have been selected to illustrate these responses. In introducing these selections, only those neurological findings associated with discernible behavioral effects have been noted along with the final diagnosis.

The clinician involved in understanding and managing these responses finds himself drawn into the general areas of geriatric medicine and psychiatry, as well as the more specific problems associated with the evaluation of the interplay of neurologic, psychiatric and environmental factors. Guideposts are needed and fortunately some do exist, especially in the work of Kurt Goldstein (3) earlier and more recently that of Weinstein and Kahn (4) on the brain-damaged patient. The contributions of these and other workers will be reviewed at a later point. The general plan will be to present clinical material illustrative of the critical points of the disease process, and to discuss the psychiatric implications of these data. In the first eight chapters the analysis is concerned, for the most part, with patients whose general mental faculties were not impaired by the stroke in an "organic" sense. In the following chapters patients with neurologic deficit severe enough to impair symbolic expression are considered. The tenth chapter deals with the results of an investigation into the immediate subjective reactions to motor deficit. In this chapter, the specific theoretical point of view developed is stated explicitly and compared with the work of other investigators.

Perhaps the title of this book might be more accurate if it were qualified by the word "some" appearing before the title as it now stands. The range of our observations does not yet permit a more inclusive account of a number of psychological problems and reactions briefly alluded to at different points in the discussion, as for example, attitudes towards dying, idiosyncratic theories as to causation of the stroke, alterations in sleep and dream patterns, subjective experiences of the aphasic patient, and a host of others.

The author wishes to acknowledge his indebtedness to Dr. Irving S. Wright and Dr. Howard Rusk, whose foresight made the project possible and who, as Principal Investigators, mapped out the problem areas to be explored; to Dr. Sigmund N. Groch who, as Medical Director of the study, displayed a remarkable dedication to the problem at hand; to Dr. Louis J. Hurwitz and Dr. Edward M. Ashenhurst who, as visitors to our shores from the National Hospital at Queen Square, London, provided original and provocative neurologic commentary, and to Miss Kathleen Monahan for her care in the organization and maintenance of the clinical records.

I also wish to express my appreciation to Dr. Arthur M. Wieder for his assistance in the psychological evaluation of the patients during the first year of the study, and to Dr. Arno Gruen who has been carrying out further psychological studies over the past two years. Finally, I want to acknowledge the helpful and much needed information provided by Phia Volkavitch and Vera Burke, the social workers on the project.

In the preparation of the manuscript I wish to acknowledge with gratitude the many helpful suggestions of Dr. Groch and Dr. Wright, as well as the editorial assistance so generously offered by my good friends, Mr. Brooks Roberts, Mrs. Laura A. Dale, and Mr. Henry Bennett.

M. U.
Ardsley, New York

CONTENTS

Behavioral Changes
in Patients
Following Strokes

CHAPTER I

THE SUBJECTIVE IMPACT

When the patient who has had a stroke is questioned soon after the onset of the illness, one often encounters a readiness and eagerness to talk about the experience. In many instances this amounts to a definite need to share and explore the emotional aftermath of an illness which may mark a dramatic turning point in the life history of the patient. Medical care and support under these circumstances are not enough. A concern with the feelings and preoccupations of the patient is essential to the therapeutic task.

Systematic questioning concerning the immediate subjective reactions associated with the onset and initial phases of the illness has been rewarding in a number of ways. When the patients are asked a few simple questions which lead into an introspective evaluation of their experience, a great deal of information concerning the operation of idiosyncratic modes of adaptation can be elicited. A sequential pattern of questioning can best bring the felt reactions of the patient into focus.

Question 1: What happened to you?

The patient, who by this time has gone through the history-taking process two or more times with the various members of the house staff, begins consciously or unconsciously to tailor his replies to what he now knows to be of interest to the physician. This question, therefore, generally elicits a factual review of the history of the present illness as the patient has experienced it.

Question 2: What did you think was happening to you?

The patients often respond with "I didn't know," but when the question is repeated several times, and accented in a way that presses for their own interpretation, there generally follows a verbalization of feelings.

Once the ice is broken in this manner and the examiner's concern for what is personal rather than what is strictly factual has transmitted itself to the patient, further exploratory questions may follow:

Question 3:   Were you frightened?

Although some degree of anxiety is the rule, any reference to it is often omitted in the patient's spontaneous account.

Question 4:   Do you have any ideas as to why this occurred?

This question discloses the balance between the patient's capacity for objective evaluation and his tendency to project blame either outward or against himself.

In the responses to these questions importance is attached to what is omitted, what is emphasized and what is misinterpreted. In addition to the immediate therapeutic benefit this type of exploratory and supportive discussion has for the patient, there is additional importance in the light it sheds on subsequent behavioral trends. Other information of interest arising out of this line of questioning concerns the possible influence of the time of occurrence of the stroke, e.g., during sleep or while awake, where the stroke occurred, whether at home or at work, in the presence or absence of other people, the rapidity of onset, the nature of the presenting symptoms, the causative theories advanced by the patient, differences involving the age factor, the role of relatives, special effect of specific motor and sensory disturbances, etc.

To the patient the stroke is always an unfamiliar disease. It arrives unheralded and unannounced and makes its presence felt with none of the usual prodromata of illness. Fever and malaise are usually absent. Pain is only occasionally present. In an age group accustomed to cardiac and hypertensive symptomatology there are few, if any, symptoms readily linked either to the heart or the increase in blood pressure. Most frequently the onset is characterized by the quiet progression of motor effects. In roughly a third of our patients the stroke occurred at night, and in only a small number of these patients did awakening occur at the time of onset of the stroke. Most often the stroke was first noticed on attempting to get out of bed. Although motor symptoms play a prominent part, the initial complaints are often couched in terms of how the limb or limbs "feel"; less often is there an immediate awareness of paralysis. Sometimes the history of a previous stroke alerts the patient to what is going on, but, because the mode of onset can be varied, it may as often not. The occurrence of a stroke in other members of the family sometimes suggests the possibility sooner than it might otherwise occur.

In most instances, however, the patients find themselves in the grip of an unfamiliar experience with few landmarks to orient them to what is happening. Depending on the individual, the initial reactions may be characterized by efforts to minimize and rationalize the developing symptoms, a vague sense of foreboding concerning something serious that is going on but without knowledge of what it is, acute anxiety and fear of impending death, and, occasionally, clear insight into the precise nature of his predicament. Stoical and courageous attitudes are more frequently noted when the patient is alone at the onset. Perhaps the urgent problem of devising a means of securing help deflects a more severe anxiety reaction. At any rate, the latter appears to be more common when the patient is in the company of other people at the onset. The most distressing immediate reactions occur when the patient is at home and amongst the members of his own family. The anxiety tends to be less acute when the patient is amongst strangers or at work. Here the impersonal elements appear to modulate the initial response. Although occasionally the anxiety takes the form of fear of impending death, it is more often linked with the idea of being a cripple and fear of helplessness.

The certain realization of having had a stroke begins to occur only after arrival at the hospital and when and if told by the admitting officer. This information is often couched in euphemistic terms such as "mild stroke." This may be enormously reassuring to the patient. Even patients with severe residual hemiplegia and other deficits often refer to their illness as a mild stroke. This makes more sense than may appear to the clinician when one contemplates the possible alternative. Often there is no clear recognition that the illness was a stroke even when efforts are made explicitly to inform the patient. The culturally-bound notions of what a stroke is and the actual disturbances experienced by the patient may be too far apart to elicit a genuine emotional response. He may report that he had a "slight shock" or "spasm" in the head, or even talk about a "hemorrhage in the head" or a "blood vessel breaking" without connecting it with the idea of a stroke.

The following examples illustrate some of these reactions:

STROKES OCCURRING DURING SLEEP

When the stroke occurs during the night sleep is generally not interrupted and there is no awareness of anything wrong until the effort is made either to leave the bed in the morning, or to get up during the night to go to the bathroom. Severe motor difficulties take the patient by surprise. When the presenting symptoms are less pronounced there may be no awareness of any deficit until the patient encounters some difficulty with finer movements while dressing, shaving or eating.

> *Case 1.* 66 year old white male. Left hemiplegia. *Diagnosis:* Thrombosis, right middle cerebral artery.
>
> "I slept well at night. When I woke up my whole left side was paralyzed. I had no feeling in it at all. I couldn't move my arm and then I found out my leg was dead. I tried to get out of bed and I couldn't make it. (What did you think was happening to you?) I couldn't imagine what it was; then it struck me I must have had a stroke or some kind of mishap during the night. I was calm. I tried to figure out what happened to me and I couldn't. (Were you frightened?) I was frightened. I didn't know what happened. The doctor came. He diagnosed it as a stroke, so my sister took me over here that night."

Comment: The patient struggled for about 20 minutes to get out of bed before he realized there was something wrong. He had been a heavy drinker over many years. His initial reaction was to connect the illness with his drinking. He commented that he had had two pints of wine and seven or eight highballs the night before. The patient had been living alone at the time of his illness. He had worked as a counterman until six years ago and since then had been on welfare. His general attitude remained one of affable acceptance of his lot. The heightened dependency status resulting from the stroke and the ensuing motor deficit was fundamentally congruent with a generally passive orientation.

Case 2. 69 year old white male. Right hemiparesis. *Diagnosis:* Thrombosis, basilar artery.

"I woke up in the morning. I couldn't use my arm. I was pretty dizzy. I tried to make a cup of coffee. I didn't know what was the matter. I staggered around the room. I made the coffee. I dropped it. Then I knew something was the matter with me. The grip was a little weak. (What did you think was the trouble?) I couldn't make out what it was. How is a man going to think when he's dizzy? (Did you think you were having a stroke?) I never gave that a thought in a million years. I lived all these years and worked so hard. A man weighing 186 pounds who is active and in good health doesn't think of it."

Comment: The patient took to his bed and began drinking. He was not admitted until two days after the onset when he was no longer able to get around by himself. He remained in bed most of the time and prevailed upon his friends to bring him whiskey. The patient had lived his life as a social isolate with a heavy reliance on alcohol. In contrast to the first patient, who sought help, this patient prevailed upon his friends to keep him supplied with alcohol.

The following patients rationalized the initial difficulties in various ways:

Case 3. 62 year old white male. Right hemiparesis. *Diagnosis:* Thrombosis, right middle cerebral artery.

"I awoke in the morning. I tried to get out of bed. My right arm and leg were paralyzed. It took me by surprise. There was no pain. I managed to walk downstairs. I wanted to cross the street and get something to eat. (What did you think was happening?) I couldn't think of anything. I thought maybe it was a cold settling on my spine. I never thought it could be a stroke. When I talked to people they looked at me in astonishment. There was something wrong with my speech."

Case 4. 65 year old white male. Left hemiparesis. *Diagnosis:* Thrombosis, branch, right middle cerebral artery.

"I got up in the morning. I went to the breakfast table. I wanted to break a piece of bread. This hand (left) was stiff and I couldn't control it. I just couldn't figure it out. I thought I had slept on it and it had become numb."

Case 5. 65 year old white male. Left hemiparesis. *Diagnosis:* Thrombosis, right internal carotid artery.

"I woke at 5. I couldn't get up. I couldn't move my left arm. I forced myself to get up and I went to the bathroom. I noticed I was going sideways. (What did you think was happening?) At first I thought something had happened to this (points to a Dupuytren's contracture of the small finger of the left hand). Ten years ago the doctor told me the hand would close on me and I thought that was what had happened. When people told me it was a stroke, I said how could it be when nothing happened to me?"

The initial awareness of illness may be associated with considerable anxiety:

Case 6. 50 year old white male. Left hemiparesis. *Diagnosis:* Thrombosis, right internal carotid artery.

"When I got dressed I knew there was something funny. I couldn't get my hand in my sleeve. I got into the car to change the parking place. As soon as I got out I fell down. I acted as though I were completely drunk. Someone looked at me and thought I was drunk. I said, 'Look, Mister, I'm not drunk; something is wrong.' I tried to get something out of my pocket and couldn't move my hand. I was frightened when they brought me in here. I was really frightened. I was scared even in the hospital."

Comment: The patient is of a worrisome and apprehensive nature, particularly in relation to illness. Seventeen years ago he experienced the sudden onset of hyperthyroidism. He felt the symptoms of nervousness and weight loss began soon after witnessing an automobile accident in which a woman was badly injured. Two thyroid operations were required within a period of three months following this incident.

Case 7. 65 year old white female. Right hemiparesis. *Diagnosis:* Thrombosis, branch, left middle cerebral artery.

"I woke at 10:30 in the morning. My hand (right) began to

tingle. The fingers felt numb. I first thought I was dying. I wanted to tell the landlady. I got to the door. I saw the landlady. I knew I was having a stroke. My leg was wobbly. My tongue was thick. My speech was affected. I couldn't talk straight."

Comment: The basis for an anxiety reaction in this patient was not connected with a fear of illness in general, but rather with a phobic reaction concerning the possibility of a syphilitic infection. She had been married in 1914 and separated from her husband three years later. Shortly after this a positive blood Wassermann was noted. She was treated for syphilis. In 1940 another 4-plus reaction was noted while hospitalized for a hysterectomy. Although it was difficult to draw her out concerning this aspect of her past, once she did begin she revealed deep feelings of guilt and shame and an anxious preoccupation with the conviction that her present illness was a syphilitic complication and represented a punitive aftermath.

When the onset is associated with sensory distress, awakening may occur during the night.

Case 8.   63 year old white male. Left hemiparesis. *Diagnosis:* Probable embolus, right middle cerebral circulation.

"It was in the middle of the night. It was a funny sensation around my heart. It felt like it was going to burst out. It went down my arm and leg. Then I found out I couldn't move my arm or leg. My vision was blurred to a certain extent. (What did you think was happening?) When I came in here they told me it was a stroke. I thought that's what it was myself. It made me worry."

STROKES OCCURRING DURING THE WAKING STATE

Some of the most poignant accounts are those of patients who are stricken while alone and who desperately strive to contact someone for help.

Case 9.   71 year old white male. Left hemiparesis. *Diagnosis:* Thrombosis, right middle cerebral artery.

"On that Saturday I got sick. I took a long walk on Riverside Drive—that was the fatal day. I walked eight miles. It was a beautiful sunny day; I walked too far, but I wasn't killing myself—I would stroll and rest. I got home about 6 o'clock. Then I walked to the 57th Street Automat for supper. Then I stood for the Perry Como TV show. I got home at 11 o'clock at night. I had walked ten miles in ten hours. I got the Sunday *Times.* From nowhere I began to feel as though I were having a mental stroke and my left arm was paralyzed. I worked on it a while, but it was absolutely dead. Then my left leg was going a little. I tottered to the toilet, getting weaker and weaker, wondering what to do. I was in a room by myself. I rested for a while and tried again to get up to leak, but I couldn't walk—I crawled. And I couldn't even do that, and I collapsed completely. I pulled myself back to bed. My mind was quite clear. I figured I couldn't get attention until Sunday. In the morning I felt a bit better. I was sort of in a daze during the night. I had no dreams. I was mostly awake; it looked to me like it was all over. I thought that was the end, or at the very least it was like a friend of mine with a stroke on the left side. In the morning the sun started to come in. I crawled to the door. I left it open so I could see anyone coming down the hall. Finally a man came along. I had written a note saying I'm sick—call the landlady, number 8 is sick. I asked him to take the paper to the landlady. She didn't come up until three in the afternoon. She thought it was in the house next door. I was lying in bed feeling a little better. She asked me if I had a doctor. She said it was not easy to get a doctor on Sunday. I figured I'd leave it up to her to get the doctor. She sent up a quart of buttermilk. About 5 the doctor came. He thought it would be better to go to the hospital and I went in on Sunday."*

Comment: The patient, a man of superior intelligence, found all of his faculties taxed by the task of establishing contact with the outside world. This served to delay a worried, anxious reaction noted later.

Other people present at the time of onset may play either a reassuring or an anxiety-provoking role. Not infrequently the patient's first clear awareness that something is wrong occurs as

---

*A very detailed and interesting account of the experiences of a stroke patient is to be found in a recently published book entitled *Stroke: A Diary of Recovery,* by Douglas Ritchie, London, 1960.

a result of the reactions of others either to his appearance or his speech.

Case 10.   70 year old white male. Paresis, left arm. *Diagnosis:* Thrombosis, branch, right middle cerebral artery.

"I was sitting in the house. My son came up to visit me. He noticed something on my face and he called my wife. I felt all right. I didn't notice anything. I started to spit and I didn't talk right. They made me more nervous than anything. They started to cry and I thought God knows what is happening to me. I asked whether my face is straight."

Comment: The fright reaction of both the son and the wife quickly induced a mounting agitated state in the patient.

Case 11.   53 year old white male. Left hemiparesis. *Diagnosis:* Thrombosis, right middle cerebral artery.

"My left leg gave in. I couldn't seem to move the left side at all. Someone came and helped me get dressed and went to the drugstore with me. I went there to get a cane. The man there said 'Mister, you've had a stroke.' (What did you think was happening to you?) I didn't know what it was. All I knew was I couldn't use my left arm and leg. When the man in the drugstore told me I got scared. I don't know why it should have happened. I don't drink and I don't go out with women."

Comment: Initially the characteristic effort to minimize or deny the significance of what he was experiencing may be noted. The pharmacist's blunt disclosure of the diagnosis evoked an acute anxiety reaction. The patient's notions concerning causality reveal the not uncommon linkage of an acute castastrophic illness with retribution and sin.

In the following examples the onset occurred at work. The reactions of the two patients are quite different:

Case 12.   53 year old white male. Paresis, left hand. *Diagnosis:* Recurrent transient intermittent ischemic episodes—right internal carotid—middle cerebral system.

"I was on the job. It was about 2 in the afternoon. I was operating a stencil machine. I started to drop the stencil in the machine when the darn tray clunked on the ground. I didn't feel it leave my hand. My left hand was numb. I sat

down and had two cigarettes. I went for coffee. How that
floor came up I don't know! I didn't feel sick. I got up myself. I got in the front of the car. I fell down again. The right
side of my face was numb. Saliva was coming and I couldn't
feel it. I started talking and I knew my speech was bad. I went
home. I didn't want to go to the hospital. My wife made me
go down to the clinic. (What did you think was happening?)
I didn't feel sick. I kind of suspected something to do with
pressure on my heart."

Comment: The patient is a man with a psychopathic and
alcoholic background. He did his best to fight off the pressure
first of his friends on the job and then of his wife to seek medical
help.

> *Case 13.* 56 year old Negro male. Right hemiparesis. *Diag-
> nosis:* Thrombosis or embolus, left middle cerebral artery.
> "It was about 4:30 in the afternoon. I was operating the
> elevator and the switchboard. There were blinding lights and
> I was lurching about as if drunk. It dawned on me to get out
> of the elevator before I hurt somebody. I went into one of the
> rooms. I called a friend to relieve me. I said it was temporary
> and I could shake it off. I was not aware of any trouble with
> my speech. I couldn't stand up. (What did you think was hap-
> pening?) I really didn't know. My eyeglasses seemed alive in
> my right hand. I could look at it in a stupid sort of way, but
> had no control over it. It seemed as if the glasses had become an
> animal or a crab. I never lost consciousness. (Were you fright-
> ened?) The only time I really got frightened was when I
> couldn't control my right hand and the glasses appeared
> animated. Other than that I wasn't panicky. I didn't know
> something was wrong with my speech until I was in the
> hospital."

Comment: In contrast with the preceding patient, there remained both a sense of his obligation to others and a reliance
on the judgment of others. The transitory illusion involving
the eyeglasses is of a type that is frequently associated with the
sudden loss of motor power and the simultaneous occurrence of
sensory changes in a limb. The movement of an inanimate object
inadvertently by the involved limb appears to originate from the

object itself as its relation to the limb and the connection of the latter to the self is not immediately perceived.

Idiosyncratic attitudes towards illness, physical handicaps and possible death can be noted in the following examples:

> *Case 14.* 58 year old Negro male. Symmetrical wasting of forearms and intrinsic muscles of both hands. Left hemiplegia. *Diagnosis:* Thrombosis, right middle cerebral artery. Myelopathy, vascular origin (old).
>
> "My first emotions were: I hoped it would be fatal. The worst thing a man can undergo is helplessness. It goes against the grain to adapt yourself to helplessness. I was not reconciled to the fact that I may be crippled. It doesn't make any difference whether I live or die. Death has no fear."

Comment: This patient had been partially disabled for at least five years prior to the onset of the stroke. Any additional handicap spelled complete helplessness and initiated a mood of resignation and indifference. He was no longer motivated to struggle against the mounting hardships he was forced to endure.

> *Case 15.* 59 year old white male. Right hemiparesis. *Diagnosis:* Thrombosis, left middle cerebral artery.
>
> "It came on so suddenly. I was driving my cab. I was at 32nd Street between First and Second Avenues when I hit a trailer truck. My right side was suddenly paralyzed. The police came. I told them I didn't know what happened. They drove me here but I signed myself out. I felt good again. There was no paralysis. (The patient returned to his cab, drove home and waited for his wife to return home from work.) The next day I lost my speech. The doctor came. He advised me to go to the hospital. (What did you think had happened to you?) I knew I had an accident. I don't know what it was. (Were you frightened?) I was scared. I didn't know whether it was a stroke or not. (Why did you sign yourself out?) I just wanted to go home. I didn't want to go there without my wife's consent. (The patient remained at home and felt all right until the afternoon of the next day.) Late that afternoon I fell to the floor. I just couldn't stand. I lost my voice. My right side was weak. (What was happening to you?) I didn't know. I went to the hospital the following day."

Comment: The personality structure of this patient was characterized by considerable immaturity. He could not tolerate separation from his wife during the period of immediate upset. He showed poor judgment in signing out of the hospital and later resisted hospitalization even when it was apparent that his wife would not be able to take care of him. Once in the hospital there was a total and obvious shift of his dependency ties to the doctors who were caring for him.

> *Case 16.* 64 year old white male. History of right hemiparesis. *Diagnosis:* Recurrent transient intermittent ischemic episodes—left internal carotid—middle cerebral system.
>
> "It was 11 or 12 at night when I started getting my paints and brushes together. I had a faraway feeling. Something, I knew, was wrong. I got up at 3 or 4 to go to the bathroom. Coming back I toppled. I had pain in my right foot and arm and I couldn't stand. I pulled myself up by my hands and knees. What the hell is this? I knew I had high blood pressure. I knew I had a stroke. My speech was involved. My friend in the apartment called the druggist. I mustered my strength. I got a stick and went to the drugstore. The druggist gave me a cane and I walked all the way here (a distance of about a mile)."

Comment: This patient was a Christian Scientist. He states that it was his belief in Christian Science that gave him the strength to get to the hospital and left him feeling certain that he would get well. He gave the following interesting account of the onset of hemianopia: "While I was walking here a hole came into my right eye. Everything seemed to be coming into it. Things went into that hole and then stopped. I don't notice it now, but it was like a round hole in the right side. Things disappeared into that hole. Now wasn't that strange? You'd think I'm crazy!"

> *Case 17.* 62 year old white female. Right hemiparesis. *Diagnosis:* Thrombosis, left middle cerebral artery. (The onset in this case occurred with loss of consciousness.)
>
> "My husband came over and found me. He thought I was dead. They woke me. I noticed a lot of people. My husband was shaking me, trying to wake me up. I noticed this hand (right) didn't move altogether. I noticed a little trouble with

my right foot. I wanted to stand near the bed but I couldn't. (What did you think was happening to you?) I was strong like an ox. All of a sudden I fell down on the floor. I didn't think. They told me. I figured this way—if I get well I'll know what happened to me. Otherwise I don't know. The doctor said it was a stroke. It didn't occur to me. (Were you frightened?) I wasn't frightened. To be frightened I wouldn't know what it is. I used to take care of a farm by myself. I was never really frightened."

Comment: The patient had been a very vigorous and hard working individual all of her life. She was an alert, outgoing and active person with very positive attitudes toward living. She endured many periods of upset earlier in her life when she emigrated to this country from Russia, and later when she and her husband encountered times of financial strain. He had been forced to stop work in recent years because of a series of heart attacks. Her attitude toward the stroke included the combined qualities of stoicism, defiance and derogation of illness.

The concept of a stroke occurring in patients in the younger age brackets is particularly difficult to grasp. More manifest anxiety appears in the initial reaction.

Case 18. 37 year old white male. Left hemiparesis. *Diagnosis:* Thrombosis, right middle cerebral artery.

"It was 9 or 10 in the morning. I was in the Automat. I tried to grab a chair with my left arm. I noticed my left arm going around the back of the chair. I got delirious. I grabbed my arm. It stopped. I finished eating. I walked to work. I had a paper under my arm. It fell. Then my leg started to go and I got a little groggy. (What did you think was happening to you?) I didn't know. I was scared as hell. I thought it was a heart attack. The doctor told someone it was a mild apoplexy. I didn't know what he meant. (Did you think you were dying?) I thought I was close to it."

Comment: The psychiatric picture was that of an inadequate personality. He was the only one of four siblings who had not succeeded in establishing an independent existence for himself. His work history was spotty and he had been unable to make any adequate heterosexual adjustment. There were two aspects to his reaction to the stroke. Initially he experienced acute anxiety almost to the point of hysteria. Once the initial excitement had abated and he no longer felt endangered, his own dependency patterns jelled into an acceptance of a state of semi-invalidism. In actuality he had a sufficient return of function to be gainfully employed.

In the case of patients who have had previous strokes recognition of what is happening may or may not occur, depending on how closely the current symptoms parallel the earlier ones.

Case 19. 57 year old white male. Right hemiparesis. *Diagnosis:* Old left middle cerebral branch occlusion (8 months ago). Recent left posterior inferior cerebellar artery occlusion.

"I was supposed to come to the brace clinic on Wednesday. I got up in the morning and was all right. Before I left I felt dizzy. I waited 15 or 20 minutes and the dizziness passed. I took the train. I got as far as the brace clinic. I fell to the left against my wife. I said 'The room is spinning.' She sat me down and one of the physicians came and took me to the emergency room. My pressure was 230. (What did you think was happening to you?) I had an idea I must have gotten another stroke. My left hand felt cold like the right hand did on the first stroke."

Comment: Apprehension concerning the possibility of a second stroke varies with the personality, intelligence and insight of the patient. In this instance hypertension had been diagnosed 20 years earlier. The patient was well aware of the possible serious implications of this, particularly after the occurrence of the first stroke. At that time, in response to anxiety, he reached out for support and reassurance. There was less anxiety following the second stroke. He appeared more resigned and accepting of his situation. He remained at home for several months and died soon thereafter during a third episode.

Case 20. 51 year old Negro male. Monoplegia, left arm. *Diagnosis:* Thrombosis, branch, right middle cerebral artery. (History of left hemiplegia five years earlier with slow recovery.)

"I noticed some weakness in my left arm. I stayed in the house. The next morning I called an ambulance. It had really gone completely bad on me. The night before I was sitting in the playground and I couldn't move my left arm. I said to my friend, 'My nerves are no good.' (What did you think was happening?) I didn't know what was happening. I was just wondering about the use of this arm. (Did you think you were having a stroke?) I had no idea it was a stroke. It was not like the first one. The idea of another stroke didn't occur to me because I could still walk on my leg."

Comment: This patient, in contrast with the preceding one, was of a very phlegmatic disposition and of limited intelligence. He had little or no genuine insight into the nature of the initial episode.

Occasionally a stroke occurs within the hospital setting. The following accounts are those of two patients who experienced a cerebral embolism while on the ward:

Case 21. 59 year old white male. Left homonymous hemianopia. *Diagnosis:* Embolus, right posterior cerebral artery. Mitral insufficiency. Auricular fibrillation.

"It happened on the ward. I said, 'Please call the doctor. I can't see.' Then all I could see was just like half a person. I could see the right side. I couldn't make people out. I saw them as a line. (What did you think was happening?) To me I didn't even have an idea it was a stroke. I couldn't make it out. Afterwards they told me. (Why do you think it happened?) Tension. I thought I was born with tension and that's the way I'll pass out. I'm filled with fear and worry and those things are not beneficial to my condition."

Case 22. 41 year old white female. Left hemiparesis. Admitted initially for cardiac complaints. *Diagnosis:* Embolism, right carotid circulation.

"It happened during supper time. I was drinking tea. The doctor was near my bed. All of a sudden I felt as if a live wire was going through my arm, as if you would turn a current on. I put my cup down. The doctor asked me what was wrong. I said, 'It's like an electric shock down my arm.' The next thing I remember, I was in a different ward. I must have blacked out. (What did you think when you awoke?) I didn't even think. I thought I heard the doctor say, 'Put her in front where she can be observed more closely.'"

CHAPTER II

STROKES AND STRESS

The wide array of variables responsible for the various forms and manifestations of the acute cerebrovascular accident are neither fully understood nor even fully known. They include instances where purely mechanical factors appear to play the predominant role, as in the case of the congenital vascular anomalies in the cerebral circulation, as well as other situations where biochemical factors and the atherosclerotic process seem to be of prime importance. It does not seem unreasonable to suppose that emotional factors may play a predisposing or pre-cipitating role. This possibility has to be assessed with caution in view of the many unknowns in the situation, the existence of similar emotional stresses in patients who do not get a stroke, and the not infrequent occurrence of the stroke in life situations that have had a positive affective coloration for many years.

The stroke population is for the most part a group of people who have from five to eight or nine decades of living behind them. They are beset by all the problems indigenous to this age group—failing physical faculties, loss of loved ones, problems of economic security, loneliness, idleness, deterioration of sensory and mental faculties, and the ever-present specter of helpless-ness or death. For most patients, therefore, it is not a difficult task to identify enduring emotional stresses arising in connection with the personal, social, physical or economic aspects of their life situation. To assess the significance of this type of wear and tear on the individual in relation to the slow progression of pathological processes in the circulatory system is a most diffi-cult task. When, as in our study, patients were questioned as to the occurrence of acute traumatic events in their lives occurring one to six months before the onset of the strokes, the answers were generally negative; or the patient simply described emotional sore points in his life existing over a period of many years. There were, however, a small group of patients, less than one per cent, where a striking temporal correlation occurred between an unusual and deeply disturbing life event and the occurrence of the stroke. What suggests itself in these instances is that the heightened emotional response operates as a precipitating factor by so altering vascular tone, hemodynamics or other related physiological factors, that there is a greater opportunity for complete closure, rupture or embolus to occur. The examples to follow illustrate this close temporal relationship between a sudden disturbance in the life situation and the occurrence of a stroke:

Case 23.   55 year old Negro female. *Diagnosis:* Thrombosis, branch, right middle cerebral artery.

On August 28, 1958, the patient was returning to New York from another city where she had visited her son who was being held on charges of homicide. Upon arrival in Grand Central Terminal she was unable to arise from her seat and noted that her face began twitching. Her tongue felt heavy and she had difficulty in talking. She was with her sister and a younger son at the time. She was very frightened. "I thought the world was coming to an end."

She was obviously reluctant to elaborate on the facts involved in her recent visit. The patient was unaware of any difficulty involving her oldest son until August 11, 1958, when she heard that he and his wife were to be divorced. The daughter-in-law had apparently left her son. She was shocked at the news. Her son had three small children and she had thought that his family situation had been stabilized. A week later the son shot his wife, who died on the way to the hospital. Several days later the patient went to see her son. The stroke occurred a little over a week after she received news of the shooting.

Both the patient and her husband were hardworking and had a strong sense of family unity. No serious difficulties had arisen with any of the three children before this. One son attends a university in the South.

Comment: The patient is a very self-contained and controlled individual who under any circumstances would find it hard to divulge much information about herself. At the time she was seen she was in the throes of a reactive depression precipitated by the plight of her son and subsequently deepened as a result of her illness.

Case 24.   50 year old white female. *Diagnosis:* Embolus, right middle cerebral artery.

This patient had a history of rheumatic fever since the age of 27. She tended to minimize both the illness and its sequelae despite the growing dyspnea on exertion and two episodes three months prior to admission of transient left-sided weakness. At that time she was examined in the cardiac clinic and was advised to enter the hospital as soon as she could arrange to for cardiac surgery (mitral commissurotomy). She postponed admission for nearly two months and capitulated only after pleading and threats by her two children. On the night prior to the planned admission she was found lying on the floor of her home, paralyzed on the left side.

The anxiety experienced by this patient in connection with the decision to undergo cardiac surgery was derived from both the realistic apprehension connected with a potentially danger-ous surgical procedure, and from the neurotic vulnerabilities inherent in her own structure. Her attitude toward any limita-tion in the past had been to drive herself all the more compul-sively. She had little tolerance for illness or disability. Cardiac surgery involved not only the realistic dangers inherent in the procedure itself, but perhaps of even greater importance, it meant the kind of realistic admission of illness for which psy-chologically she was completely unprepared. The dangers of facing the world without her facade of inviolability and the illusion of enduring strength and youthfulness were very real to this patient. Her anxieties were deepened not only by the limitations imposed by her illness, but also by the fact that both her children were rapidly growing apart from her and the chances of rebuilding an independent life were waning. (Her husband had died two years earlier.)

In the next two examples unusual and distressing experiences occurred shortly before the stroke. They were less dramatic and intense than in the preceding examples, although the temporal relationships remain suggestive of their possible role in the occurrence of the stroke.

Case 25. 51 year old white male. *Diagnosis:* Thrombosis, right middle cerebral artery.

In this instance the patient spontaneously introduced his preoccupation with the traumatic event into the account of his present illness. "It started off with two fingers, then my arm and the left side of my face, and then my speech. In the middle of the night I wanted to go to the bathroom. I couldn't get up. (What did you think was happening?) I didn't think. I felt funny. Could this be brought about by a shock? Because two weeks before I had a shock. My daughter lives in Tucson. (Patient begins to cry.) She was giving birth. They called us and said the child was critical. My wife and I flew out. For two weeks we were under a big strain. One of the baby's lungs hadn't opened. Two weeks later I was feeding the baby. Suddenly she seemed to choke. I felt panicky. I blew into her mouth. I was alone at the time. It was after that that I began to feel weak in my fingers. This started out there when I was worried. My daughter has asthma."

Comment: At several points in his account the patient experienced what appeared to be bouts of forced crying, particularly when referring to his daughter and grand-daughter. The trip to Arizona filled him with dread. The feeding incident was actually a minor episode but it precipitated a torrent of anxiety and almost psychotic ideas of guilt. Another, but unrelated source of tension was his fear of being placed on night duty in his job as a postal clerk. His personality pattern was basically schizoid.

Case 26. 63 year old white female. *Diagnosis:* Rheumatic carditis, mitral stenosis and insufficiency, auricular fibrillation. Probable embolus, basilar artery.

The patient had been under treatment for rheumatic heart disease for a number of years. She had a transitory cerebral accident two years ago. She was hospitalized for three weeks and then resumed her regular responsibilities at home. In recounting her initial subjective reactions to the present episode she stressed her fear of helplessness rather than of dying. Her fear was not of death itself, but of a lingering death. She tended to be somewhat controlled and self-contained.

One week before the onset of her illness the patient received a letter from a nephew in Israel. The letter included a lengthy description of the deaths of her sister and of numerous other members of her family in Germany during the war. The patient had known that her family had been wiped out, but she had not received any letters from anyone abroad since 1931. This letter was the first personal and detailed report of what had occurred. The receipt of the letter, much to her own surprise, released a floodgate of feeling. Just the recall of the incident evoked an agitated, tearful state.

Comment: The general feeling about this patient's life is one of bleakness and lack of fulfillment. The husband is weak, inadequate and somewhat paranoid. Early in her marriage she remained childless because of the need to work and supplement the meager earnings of her husband. Later on she was unable to have children. Her real emotional investments remained centered about the various members of her family in Europe despite the many years of separation. The letter from Israel brought the reality of their demise home to her and cut through any remaining illusions about their fate. Her feelings about living are summed up in the following remarks to the examiner: "I'm not afraid of dying. I have nobody. I'm all alone with my husband and he can't do nothing for me."

The following two protocols are given at greater length as they represent the more usual balance of influences—psychological, social, economic and physical—converging upon the patient destined to have a stroke.

> *Case 27.*   53 year old white male of German extraction. He was admitted to the hospital April 4, 1957. *Diagnosis:* Thrombosis, right middle cerebral artery.
>
> The patient was born and educated in Germany, completing the equivalent of two years of college. Both parents are still living. There is one younger sibling. The father was a tool maker. He is described by the patient as very strict but having a wonderful heart. He left his family and came to this country in 1931, hoping to get into the hotel business.
>
> The patient met his wife in this country. He was obviously reluctant to talk about the relationship. The marriage terminated in divorce after sixteen years, apparently on his wife's

initiative. Their personalities were quite different. "She was always happy and always ready to help others. I was always worried. I would worry about what the next day would bring. When I wasn't working I was restless and nervous." Further cause for conflict was the antagonism between his mother-in-law and himself. He characterized her as domineering and mean. There was one child, a son, who went to live with the mother when the marriage broke up in 1947. He has not seen his child since the separation.

After coming to this country he had a succession of jobs as a waiter and had worked himself up into a number of responsible positions in some of the leading restaurants. Soon after the termination of his marriage he began to have complaints referable to his heart and was told he had "cardiac asthma." From that time on physical incapacity began to interfere with his ability to work. He felt embittered by what he regarded as unfair and arbitrary discrimination by employers because of his cardiac ailment. Last November, after working as a cashier at a well-known restaurant for six months, he was suddenly given notice. He became depressed and soon was again hospitalized for cardiac complaints.

He appeared depressed during his hospital stay but denied any suicidal preoccupations. His only motivation centered about the effort to gather enough funds together from welfare and other agencies to return to Germany.

Comment: With the advent of the stroke the patient seemed to have lost any remaining ability to struggle to maintain an independent existence. Passive, dependent traits came to the fore, pushing toward the establishment of an anaclitic existence. He did not resign from life so much as from the struggle to compete and provide for himself. In line with this there was some effort to maximize his disability. The stroke in this case touched off a reactive depression which had been gathering momentum over the past ten years, beginning with the separation from his wife and the onset of cardiac complaints. He did manage to return to Germany and died there a short time later.

Case 28. 72 year old white male. Diagnosis: Thrombosis, right middle cerebral artery.

This patient's account of his life can best be given in his own words:

"I was born in Liverpool. In England you might say I was more of an executive. I came here in May, 1930. I came here as a mechanic and I went to live with my sister and brother-in-law, who was a builder. I worked as a tradesman. In England I was an executive in my own line, which was that of an electrician. When I was there my sister sent me a ticket to the States just to look around. The Consul couldn't give me a visitor's visa—he gave me an immigration visa. I decided to stay. During the depression years I took a job with a millionaire looking after an estate. Then I came to New York and fooled around at odd jobs—as a handyman, mechanic, and engineer, until I got sick in 1947. I had a prostate gland operation in 1947, then I went back to my original trade as a furniture finisher. My English experience and my American experience made me quite a craftsman. I worked more or less at odd jobs until I got the stroke.

"My father was a Swedish sailor. He went to sea. He was a very good sailor. He took pride in his ship. He broke his leg and it was set badly by the captain and had to be amputated. He came to Liverpool and married an English woman. They had one daughter. He was a big, heavy, strong man. His wife died and he opened a sailors' boarding house. He sent to Sweden for a cook. My mother came as the cook. She was a country girl. She married my father. They had 11 children. Two died. I was the third. There were three boys, then three girls, and then three boys. We were brought up very well. We weren't forbidden to smoke. As a result none of us was smokers. Things didn't go too well for the family. We opened a store, but nothing worked out too well. My father became a shipping agent. My eldest brother was a clerk with a sugar merchant. My second brother was a bit on the wild side. He couldn't hold a job and he finally went to sea. I learned a trade as a furniture polisher when I was about 13 or 14. Then I went into the electrical business. My family needed a steady job. I stayed on the job 14 years and became a top executive. My eldest brother got in with a religious protestant group. Finally he lost his job. For two or three years he was helped by my father. Finally the family separated. My mother felt the children should get a better break. We were living in a slum district. She had just had enough, I guess, with all these children. My father still wanted more—he was a very sexy man.

He would play around if he had the chance. He had a way with women, like all Scandinavians. I went with my mother, the others with my father. They liked my father better. I just liked my mother better. She had to have somebody and I had a steady job. Then my sister came to New York. Another sister came over and married a Dane in Ohio. I took my younger brothers and sister and mother and went to live in Liverpool. My father went to Sweden. I managed to take care of the kids. My mother took sick. With all this fighting her mind began to weaken. She hated England. She felt the English women were persecuting her. She got a sort of persecution complex and wanted to go home to Sweden. So I sent her home to Sweden. I sent the younger boy to her. Every two weeks I sent her an allowance. My younger sister became the housekeeper for us. My sister was an emancipated woman—a suffragette. Then came the war. My younger brother joined right away. He got his knee shattered. I was called into the mechanized transport."

(Patient was asked further about his parents.)

"They were easy-going. I realized they had had enough of each other. My mother had had enough. My father would have gone on having children. He would have been willing to have stayed in the slum district. She had ambitions for the children. I was in the army four years. She died two years after I came back. She was always sick. She had ulcers of the stomach. Going back to Sweden was the right thing for her. Her mind cleared and she had no more mental trouble. I never saw her again. I took everything as a matter of fact, like the way I'm taking my illness. She died, and then my father died on the way to Ellis Island. He was a little over 60. My younger sister made a good marriage. So now I wanted to come over here to America. I was 43 years old. I was housekeeper for my two younger brothers. I had become quite a good cook."

(There was a marked withdrawal response from the patient when he was asked to talk about his own sexual development and experiences.)

"I've got to know you better. Maybe when you do something for me, I'll do something for you. Anyway, I don't see how that will help me."

(Patient was asked about his plans.)

"I'm anxious to go. My pension checks will be coming in. I don't know what's happening in my room. As long as I'm

feeling good, I'm satisfied. I can come in for the tests. I don't
have any plans. I have a number of inventions. They are de-
vices that could be manufactured and might make millions.
I write to many people. I'm writing the story about my experience. My life is all planned for me. I like money, but I don't
worry about it. I keep in good health and do whatever turns
up. (He was encouraged to talk about his inventions.) They
are practical inventions. I used to be a painter. I invented an
extension for the paint brush. It's over ten years and I'm still
working on it. I have a patent. Then a sponge extension and
a sand scraper. Then a sponge for washing—that's in the domes-
tic field. All kinds of attachments with rollers for housecleaning.
None have been marketed. I found out they are a bunch
of crooks and all they want is your ideas. They want them for
nothing. I never thought businessmen could be so dishonest.
I have been thinking now of Good Will Industries—I could
use my ideas for the handicapped. Then I will show them
anything I've got."

Comment: Despite his protest to the contrary, his recent illness had left the patient quite shaken. There are evidences of
grandiose and paranoid trends in his make-up, but they do not
overshadow the healthier aspects of his personality. His life
has been characterized by the absence of close relationships with
anyone outside of his own family, the failure to establish any
adequate heterosexual adjustments, and the reliance on his inner
resources in the form of his imagination and inventiveness to
provide a source of satisfaction and gratification. In his initial
response to the stroke he was able to surrender all responsibility
for himself first to his landlady and then to the hospital author-
ities. His preoccupation with his inventions as a potential source
of sudden wealth and recognition was intensified in a somewhat
desperate manner in the wake of his illness.

CHAPTER III

REACTIVE FEATURES

In the pages to follow, examples will be given of reaction patterns to the stroke experience that vary from realistic integration of the experience to psychotic deterioration. These patterns are a function of the extensiveness of the brain damage, the strengths and weaknesses of the premorbid personality structure and the possibilities and limitations of the patient's current life situation. Given these three sets of determinants, there can be expected, and actually do occur, enormous individual differences in response in the weeks and months following the stroke. As noted previously, some indication is often given in the initial account of the patient's subjective reactions of the direction the adaptive responses are taking, e.g., toward realistic integration of the experience, toward minimization of the event and denial of disability, or toward an increased emphasis on the resultant disability with accentuation of dependency strivings.

The following general statements concerning reactive states are offered with the qualification that they represent very broad generalizations in an area where only accurate knowledge of the individual patient provides a dependable guidepost.

(1) *The most critical determinant is the presence or absence of a sufficient degree of brain damage to result in diffuse functional impairment with resultant defects in orientation, memory, judgment and all aspects of cognitive functioning.* To the extent that diffuse brain damage exists, the adaptive processes are reorganized at the very concrete level of enabling the individual to cope with the prevailing environmental stimuli so as to dispose immediately of any disturbing stimulus. The adaptive processes engage with the most superficial aspects of the situation and do not engage in depth with the total experience. Hence, to the

outside observer the patient appears lacking in insight, irrational or child-like. When recovery does not take place, disposition often requires either psychiatric hospitalization or nursing home placement. When these patients are discharged home to the care of relatives they are often very difficult to manage.

Concreteness of thought, unawareness of illness and disorientation are illustrated in the following interview:

Case 29.   81 year old white male. Right hemiparesis. *Diagnosis:* Thrombosis, left middle cerebral artery.
Q.   Where are you now?
A.   Home.
Q.   What kind of place is this?
A.   This is all right.
Q.   What is the name of this place?
A.   They call it a shop.
Q.   Where is it?
A.   Downtown on Essex Street.
Q.   Why did you come to this place?
A.   Why did you come? That's a question! It's ridiculous!
Q.   Where is the last place you lived in?
A.   Downtown.

In the next patient, delusional features were part of the confused state. Psychiatric hospitalization was necessary.

Case 30.   77 year old white female. Right hemiparesis. *Diagnosis:* Thrombosis, left internal carotid artery.

The interview took place at the bedside, the patient seated in a chair. She is a little old lady with a shrunken appearance. As the examiner approached she spontaneously remarked:

"They're going to arrest me. I didn't do nothing out of the way. I'm just peaceful and quiet here."
Q.   Where are you now?
A.   Here. Here, the Salvation Army at Fort Hamilton. Aren't they awful people to hold me here? You don't belong to the Salvation Army. I don't know your name.

(There was a chair near the patient with a blanket folded upon it. The examiner sat down, thus concealing the blanket. The patient immediately cried out):

"Did they steal the blanket? They took it away!"
Q.   What is today's date?

A. Saturday.

Q. What year?

A. '96 I guess.

Q. What month?

A. (Patient counted the months from January to November. The actual month was April.)

Q. Why are you here?

A. I was arrested. They brought me here from Fort Hamilton.

Q. Where are you now?

A. Fort Hamilton.

Q. What is your age?

A. (Patient gave her name.)

Q. How old are you?

A. About 42. I might be 43 or 44. Something like that.

Q. Are you married?

A. Eight or nine or ten years.

Q. What is your husband's name?

A. D. - - - -

Q. Do you have any children?

A. I had two. One died and one lived. He's about 20 now.

Q. What is this place?

A. Fort Hamilton.

Q. Who are these people? (Other patients.)

A. I don't know. I just came here today. (Patient admitted three months ago.)

Q. Why are there beds here?

A. It's a hospital.

Q. I thought you said it's the Salvation Army.

A. No. It's a hospital. It's for the sick.

Q. Are you sick?

A. No, thank God! They took me here! The cops arrested me.

Toward the end of the interview the patient showed increasing awareness of the hospital surroundings. She took the medicine offered by the nurses in an automatic way. She did, however, continue to remain confused about the reason for her being there and frequently reiterated her delusional ideas about being arrested. Her experience of time seemed to be telescoped a decade or two into the past. She was unaware of the obvious discrepancies in her responses.

The following patient showed a confusional amnesic state during her hospitalization. She was discharged home to the care of her husband and daughter. As the organic picture cleared to some extent, depressive elements came into greater prominence, ultimately necessitating psychiatric hospitalization.

Case 31. 60 year old white female. Partial cortical blindness. *Diagnosis:* Thrombosis, left posterior cerebral artery.

Q. What happened to you?
A. Nothing that I know.
Q. Why are you here?
A. To tell you the truth, I don't know.
Q. Are you sick?
A. Who am I supposed to be? What's my name?
Q. What is your name?
A. I heard someone say Mrs. P - - -. Mike P - - -, that's my husband.
Q. What hospital are you in?
A. The name I don't know. It's supposed to be on Sixth Avenue.
Q. What street is it on?
A. Sixth Avenue and 1st Street. To tell the truth, I don't remember a thing.
Q. What's today's date?
A. Today is supposed to be Saturday.
Q. What month?
A. You're going too far into history.
Q. What year?
A. I really don't know. Everything is different than it used to be.
Q. How long have you been here?
A. Too long. I don't remember.
Q. Where were you born?
A. Poland.
Q. What year?
A. When I took sick I was 55 years old.
Q. What year were you born?
A. You mean when I took sick?
Q. No, what year were you born?
A. I remember my husband used to tell me I was 55.
Q. Do you have any children?

A.   No. I had. I know I had. I don't know. I used to
have S - - -, H - - -, my husband's sister's children.

Q.   Who is the President?

A.   If he's still alive—what do you call him? He's a sick
man. Is the President still alive?

Q.   How old are you?

A.   I'm supposed to be 55. They say I'm an invalid.

Q.   Who?

A.   Oh, the people around me.

The outstanding feature was the marked uncertainty in
response to questions concerning personal identity. She exhibited at times apparent unawareness of illness in addition
to her orientation difficulties for person, time and place. She
did not complain of, nor was she apparently upset by her
visual difficulties, but in response to leading questions she
agreed that she could not see well.

The patient was seen three months following her discharge
from the hospital. At that time the daughter indicated that on
her mother's return home she seemed in better contact and
more related to her surroundings than at any time during her
hospital stay. The patient showed an impaired sense of direction
and seemed to get lost in her own apartment. The daughter
also noted that her mother had become increasingly depressed,
cried easily and complained frequently about nightmares. She
complained that her whole left side felt numb and frozen. "I'm
alive and yet I'm cold. I would like to walk and jump into the
river. I hate myself. If I could destroy myself today I'd be
very happy. I'm no good to anybody. I think I've lived long
enough. I'm talking crazy. Many times I thought of destroying
myself, but the water is too cold."

The daughter also indicated a growing suspiciousness on her
mother's part toward her husband. She accused her husband of
trying to poison her and of having another woman.

The patient had a recurrent hallucinatory experience involving her sister-in-law. "I dream too much. Everything is
real to me. Is it possible for a dead woman to come and dress
you? My sister-in-law came to help me get dressed, to look
like a lady. I heard her voice like I hear your voice."

Comment: An underlying depressive reaction of many years'
duration is seen emerging into focus, precipitated by the recent

illness, the resultant physical deficits and the inability to return to her former independent way of life.

(2) *In the absence of diffuse cerebral dysfunction the next most important determinant of the behavioral response is the severity and duration of the resultant physical disability.* The deficits most frequently encountered are the aphasic disturbances and motor loss involving one or more extremities.

In the following two clinical examples, the reactions of two patients both in their sixties and both highly motivated to return to their premorbid way of life are compared. In the first, a hemiparesis occurred which was transient. In the second, a hemiplegia persisted with little or no change. No intellectual impairment was noted in either instance.

> *Case 32.* 63 year old white male. Transient hemiparesis. *Diagnosis:* Thrombosis, left middle cerebral artery.
>
> Patient had a history of good health until nine years prior to admission, when he was hospitalized and anticoagulated for a thrombosis in his right leg. Three years prior to admission diabetes was discovered. One half hour prior to admission he experienced a dizzy spell while on the subway. He lost consciousness and awoke to find himself in the hospital. He had a right hemiparesis which cleared soon after admission.
>
> In the hospital he appeared eager for contact, optimistic, and engaged in jocular exchanges with the examiner. He spoke with confidence about his recovery and return to work. He had a tendency to express himself in positively tinged cliches such as: "If you don't bother trouble it doesn't bother you," or "Health comes first."
>
> The patient made an uneventful recovery and did return to work.

> *Case 33.* 67 year old white male of Armenian extraction. Right hemiplegia. *Diagnosis:* Thrombosis, left middle cerebral artery.
>
> Prior to his illness the patient worked part time as a tailor. He was born in Armenia and has been in this country since the age of 30. He has never married. When questioned about this his eyes became tearful and he told of a romance in the old country some 40 years before. He had been deeply in love with a girl who died suddenly of meningitis.

In recent years his interests have centered about music and reading. He played both the violin and the guitar. He enjoyed spending time at an Armenian social club to which he belonged.

He verbalized his reaction to the realization that he had had a stroke as follows: "It wasn't easy. I am a cripple now. I think about my future. Now I am an old man. I try everything to save myself; my arm is not good." On the ward he was observed constantly to exercise his hand and arm. As time passed with little or no change, he became increasingly discouraged and more and more began to express feelings of hopelessness and futility. The prospect of discharge to a nursing home intensified the depressive reaction.

(3) *The next important determinant of the behavioral response is the life situation to which the patient is likely to return.* This is a very heterogeneous category made up of many components. Included here are all the residual sustaining elements in the individual's life. What are the gratifications remaining in terms of relatedness to work, family, friends, or the pursuit of purely individual sources of pleasure and satisfaction? When the two preceding patients are compared, the first returned to a life situation from which no essential ingredient was lacking. The second returned to a life situation drastically more circumscribed and limited, even by comparison with an already shrunken sphere of activity.

In the following two patients the life situations were altered in contrasting ways by essentially similar residual deficits.

Case 34. 70 year old white female. Expressive aphasia. *Diagnosis:* Thrombosis, left middle cerebral artery.

This patient exhibited a nearly total expressive aphasia throughout her stay in the hospital. She did not appear to have any difficulty in understanding the speech of others. Reading was not impaired. Attempts at speech resulted in the perseveration of a few unintelligible symbols. She appeared alert and eager for contact.

Prior to her illness she had been living a completely independent existence. Arrangements were made prior to discharge for her to live with a close and devoted friend of long standing. When this patient was seen for a follow-up six months after discharge from the hospital it was apparent that the arrangement had worked out satisfactorily for both parties. The friend described the patient as cheerful, alert and active. She was able to care for her own needs and handle her share of the housework. The aphasic disorder was essentially un-modified.

Case 35. 60 year old white male. Expressive aphasia. *Diagnosis:* Thrombosis, left middle cerebral artery.

As in the preceding case, this patient was capable of under-standing spoken words and of reading. He began to experi-ence a reactive depression in the early phase of his illness. He appeared listless, apathetic and by gesture indicated his resig-nation and futility.

The patient was born in Russia and emigrated to this country in 1908. He was graduated from a mid-Western uni-versity in 1917 with a degree in civil engineering. He was married the following year. He was described by his wife as "intelligent, resourceful and philosophical." After a variegated earlier work history he began to employ his linguistic and journalistic abilities in earning his livelihood. He was able to earn enough money from translation work and free-lance writing to support his wife and himself. He was employed by the Government during the last war as a language consultant, being an expert in German and French, in addition to Russian.

The depression lifted a little after speech therapy got under way. This was more a response to the supportive and encour-aging impact of the relationship rather than any objective im-provement in speech.

The depressive reaction deepened following his discharge from the hospital. He was unable to resign himself to the en-forced idleness and the physical impossibility of continuing his journalistic endeavors. A second stroke occurred six months after discharge followed by a gradual downhill course.

Comment: In the first instance (Case 34) the life situation was altered in a way that, for the patient, compensated for the residual aphasic deficit. In the second instance (Case 35) the same residual handicap dominated the return of the patient to a life situation that otherwise remained unaltered.

(4) In evaluating the influence of premorbid personality fac-

*tors on the subsequent behavioral response of the patient, two con-
tradictory aspects are immediately noted. In one sense, the premorbid personality is all-important. It forms the nexus out of
which all subsequent adaptive responses arise. On the other hand,
any conventional classification of premorbid personality patterns
is quite useless as a basis for predicting either healthy or pathological modes of integrating the impact of the stroke.* Patients
with a pre-existing schizophrenic pattern may move through the
entire experience without any basic changes becoming evident.
Others with a similar or borderline structure may flare up into
an acute episode. Most commonly what occurs is an accentuation
of underlying trends of either a positive or negative quality.
Thus, patients may move towards states of more outspoken
benevolence, tolerance and appreciation or, conversely, irascibility, suspiciousness, dissatisfaction and intolerance. In some
instances attitudes and reactions diametrically opposed to prevailing trends in the premorbid personality come into focus.
Emotional lability, often seen in these patients, is difficult to
evaluate because of the uncertain role of possible pathologic
processes. In short, the many variables—social, psychological and
physical—entering into the final adaptive response dilute the
possible prognostic importance of a knowledge of the life history
of the individual. In no way, however, does that fact gainsay the
importance of this knowledge in the management and treatment
of maladaptive responses when these do occur.

In the following example a patient with a markedly deviant
premorbid personality structure had a stroke with no lasting
residual effects. The occurrence of the stroke neither significantly
impaired nor affected the pre-existing compensatory mechanisms.

Case 36. 55 year old white male. Transitory brain stem
signs. *Diagnosis:* Thrombosis, basilar artery.

The onset of the stroke occurred with vertigo, nausea and
ataxia which gradually cleared after admission to the hospital.
At the time of his admission he was extraordinarily dirty and
foul smelling. Speech was animated but difficult to understand
because of a rapid-fire staccato-like type of delivery.

Patient is the only child of his mother's second marriage.
His half sister, who is now in her 70's, lives in Paris where the

patient lived until the age of 15. He describes himself as a "nervous" though physically healthy child who led an uneventful existence until the age of seven, when he began to attend school. Although he was a good student, he was expelled from one school and transferred to another because of his "mischievous" behavior. He was derided by his peers who called him "crazy" because he talked aloud and out of turn, jumped and ran about his classroom. As a child, the patient delighted in "teasing." He rang doorbells and played other similar pranks, apparently reserving these attentions for the adults in his environment. He had one friend at school but did not continue this association beyond the classroom. He did not engage in sports, spent most of his time reading novels or day-dreaming. These interests led him in his late teens to write a novel which he tried, unsuccessfully, to have published. Following this he continued to write songs and stories about bandits and detectives, but no longer sought recognition.

The patient describes his father as a strict disciplinarian who wanted him to learn a trade and cautioned him that "too much imagination will make you crazy." The patient's mother worked throughout his childhood and adult life as a milliner and seamstress. He describes her as "easy to get along with" and "easy to talk with." Although she shared her husband's occupational ambitions for the patient, he felt closer to her than to his father.

Following the completion of his sixth year of schooling, the patient and his parents traveled to Spain, where his father taught languages. In 1916 the family emigrated to the United States, returning to France five years later. The patient was then able to secure a job as a clerk, work which apparently represented the height of his ambition. He left his job in 1930 when his parents decided to return to the United States to take up permanent residence. He lived with his parents in New York City until their deaths, his father at the age of 86 in 1938 and his mother in 1943 at the age of 82. Since that time the patient has lived alone in a furnished room. He has worked at his present job as a messenger for the past 13 years.

His life has in general been devoid of meaningful relationships since the death of his parents, except for a kind of childlike attachment to an older woman, a friend of his mother's who stepped in and exercised a caretaker role in his life. He gives as the reason for his seclusiveness and inability to pursue other than menial jobs his fear of people and shyness.

Although the patient has had trouble with his vision since childhood and has had impaired hearing since the age of 13, the stroke, which caused his admission to Bellevue, was the first major illness of his life. He appeared to be both puzzled and frightened by it.

Psychological testing revealed a full-scale IQ of 120 and a verbal IQ of 132. Projective studies indicated a long-standing schizophrenic process associated with stable compensatory mechanisms. His premorbid mode of existence continued unchanged following his discharge from the hospital.

The next patient had three depressive episodes, one requiring shock treatment, prior to the stroke. Although left with a motor deficit there was no recurrence of the depressive episode.

Case 37. 52 year old white male. Flaccid paralysis right hand. *Diagnosis:* Thrombosis, left middle cerebral artery.

The patient is a married man who earned his living as a baker. He has four children ranging in age from 14 to 25. One child had a congenital deformity of the spine, necessitating operation. There is also difficulty with an older son who was recently expelled from college because of gambling. The patient describes himself as sensitive, worrisome and chronically depressed. Five years ago he was hospitalized for a depression and received 12 shock treatments. One year ago he received psychiatric treatment at an out-patient clinic for another depressive episode. He also recalls a period of depression following the death of his mother eight years ago.

His reaction to the present illness was marked by anxiety and mild depression, both of which diminished following discharge. Although he considered the idea, he did not feel the need for any further psychiatric treatment at the time of his discharge.

Accentuation of paranoid trends is not uncommonly seen in the older age group.

Case 38. 75 year old white female. Left hemiparesis. *Diagnosis:* Thrombosis, right middle cerebral artery.

This patient has been living by herself for the past 15 years following the death of her husband. On the day of admission she felt well until she began to prepare breakfast. Then she experienced the sudden onset of dizziness, confusion and vomiting. When first seen she was garrulous, agitated and centered all of her comments around a neighbor who she felt was persecuting her. She was asked to give an account of the onset of her illness.

"I have a peculiar story to tell you. I have a neighbor who has done everything to make life miserable. She hounded me, breaking into my room and stealing my things. She broke the chain on my door. That's the reason I don't want to go back to the room. She has spit on me and called me a sucker. My health is being ruined. I had to go to the police. She resented anybody being nice to me. She is 84. I'm entitled to live the rest of my life without her torturing me."

Comment: Whatever the reality of the provocation concerning the neighbor referred to, the fact appears to be that the patient has incorporated this into an underlying trend in her own personality. She is a very lonely woman whose ego supports fell away with the death of her husband and the loss of her former economic security. She now appears as a seclusive and pathetic figure whose fear of the external world is expressed in the anxiety and concern she shows about her neighbor. The vanity and narcissism in her make-up were revealed in her excessive use of cosmetics and a fanciness in dress, all rather inappropriate to her age and general appearance. Her preoccupation with the annoyances and interferences by this old neighbor is the final common pathway through which she is handling the anxieties and frustrations stemming from her many real problems in life. When seen in the follow-up clinic the paranoid trends were markedly subdued and the old neighbor was regarded more as a nuisance than a persecutor.

More frequently the paranoid reaction is more diffuse and tends to include some aspect of the hospital milieu.

Case 39. 75 year old white female. Left hemiparesis. *Diagnosis:* Thrombosis, right middle cerebral artery.

The patient is a petite talkative woman who rambles on in a garrulous manner:

"I feel kind of weak. Six weeks ago yesterday, I came here. Do you speak French? I can go wash in the washroom but they won't let me, these colored girls. They're terrible. It's not Bellevue like it used to be. They think they can rule Bellevue. Oh, no, not yet! There's too much girl-friend and boy-friend business going on. They brought all of Harlem here. The hospital isn't clean the way it used to be."

The paranoid ideas concerning the Negro personnel, the deterioration of the hospital and the hints at clandestine sexual activities persisted during the hospital stay. When this patient was seen in the follow-up clinic three and six months following discharge, occasional anti-Negro and anti-Semitic remarks would be made, but the patient seemed more aware of their inappropriateness and some effort would be made to cover up her comment.

Her life situation was in many respects similar to the previous patient's. Her husband had died 14 years before, and she too had once been in much better social and economic circumstances. In contrast, however, she had two married children and did not live alone but with a younger sister. In this instance, the occurrence of the stroke appears to have transformed long-standing xenophobic attitudes into delusional paranoid trends.

In the next patient oppositional trends and defensiveness in the premorbid personality gave rise to a reactive mood of irascibility, defensiveness and impatience.

Case 40. 52 year old white male. Right hemiparesis. *Diagnosis:* Thrombosis, branch, left middle cerebral artery.

Patient appeared antagonistic and annoyed in the interview situation. He would start the conversation with the sharply worded demand or accusation: "I want to get out of here," or, in a disgusted tone, "They tell me I won't be able to do electrical work again." He volunteered no spontaneous information about himself and his answers tended to be curt and non-informative. The only area in which he spoke with some openness was his work as a radio electrician. He at first denied that he was married. Later, suspecting that the examiner knew about his marriage, he spoke evasively about having been married and separated and having two children. When his guardedness and belligerence were pointed out, there was a momentary expression of remorse, followed soon after by further expressions of annoyance or vituperative comments extending to the entire hospital staff. At one point he was able to verbalize his reaction to the interview by hinting that he thought the examiner was out to prove that he was crazy. The clinical impression of a basically immature and dependent individual with diffuse paranoid defensiveness was corroborated by psychological studies:

"This patient shows defective functioning on tasks of verbal abstraction which appears to be a function of an overwhelming oppositional trend rather than a direct reflection of a defect in abstract attitude. This interpretation is reinforced by the finding that in non-verbal tasks of abstraction where failure is even more intimately associated with organic deficit, he performs not only well, but best in relation to his other abilities. There is evidence of organic impairment in the form of loss of control in planning, ordering, attention and of disorganization of perceptual patterns when under tension."

In the next patient premorbid psychopathic trends resulted in the functional superimposition of speech and motor difficulties upon transient deficits in these areas for secondary gain.

Case 41. 56 year old white male. Left hemiplegia. *Diagnosis:* Basilar artery stenosis.

The onset began with periods of apnea associated with pain down the left side and the development of a left hemiplegia. When first seen the patient presented an expressionless facies, absence of tongue movements, a left flaccid hemiplegia and a sharply defined left homonymous hemianopia. Initially, no speech could be elicited. He is a right-handed individual. The EEG showed diffuse abnormality with 4-6 cycle per second waves replacing the alpha.

At the end of the first week in the hospital hysterical features were noted. He showed a "belle indifference" in regard to the condition of his left arm. (There were no neurologic evidences of paralysis.) He showed a peculiar type of verbal responsiveness. He was able to respond appropriately, but only after long hesitation and when a response occurred it was confined to one or two words. There was no receptive difficulty in speech. He did not spontaneously move either extremity on the left side. In contrast to most hemiplegics who, with change of position use the good arm to rearrange the paralyzed arm, this patient effected elaborate changes of position without making the slightest effort to bring the weak arm into a more comfortable position by using his good arm. Muscle testing on the weak side brought antagonistic muscles into play very prominently so that it was apparent that the patient had a good deal more strength in that arm than he was either aware of or cared to indicate. It was also of interest that as the speech difficulty noted above began to recede a peculiarity was noted in his writing. He printed his words carefully and evenly, and formed sentences without any difficulty, but used absolutely no punctuation.

Prior to his illness the patient led an isolated and shift-less existence working sporadically at odd jobs and spending most of what he earned on drink. Although he came of a large family he had long since severed all ties with his siblings. He was elusive and cagey in revealing any significant details of his own past. From other sources it was learned that there was at least one period of imprisonment from 1948 to 1951. His general pattern was to travel about the country during the summer and return to the Men's Shelter in New York for the winter. It is worth noting in this connection that he was admitted in February and, although most of the initial indications of organic disorder disappeared in three to four weeks, the hysterical features persisted until June, resulting in prolongation of his hospital stay until the warm weather had set in.

Among our patients lability of mood has been associated with aphasic disturbances and depressive reactions.

Case 42. 53 year old white female. Right hemiparesis. Dysphasia. *Diagnosis:* Thrombosis, left middle cerebral artery.

The patient showed some evidence of expressive and receptive speech difficulty on admission. When she did speak, it was in a slow, hesitant, uninflected manner. In addition to the recent stroke, there was a mild post-encephalitic Parkinsonism, hypertension and diabetes.

On the ward she generally appeared sad and morose. Speech improved considerably in the first four weeks following admission. From time to time in the interview situation there would be sudden episodic bouts of agitation and crying. These seemed to be precipitated by the examiner's reference to any of the many troubled areas in her life past and present—e.g., her desertion by her husband 30 years ago, the onset of encephalitis soon after her marriage at the age of 18, the recent death of a sister, etc.

The extreme reactions gradually disappeared and were not a permanent part of the picture when the patient was seen six months and a year after discharge. There did remain, however, a discernible tendency to over-react emotionally in relation to both pleasant and unpleasant feelings. When questioned about the excessive reaction noted in the hospital, the patient said she was aware at the time that, although she felt sad and discouraged, she did not feel as unhappy as the frequent episodes of uncontrollable agitation seemed to indicate. She was mystified by the intensity of her own reactions.

CHAPTER IV

DEPRESSIVE REACTIONS

Although reactive in nature, the depressions experienced by stroke patients differ in several respects from the usual type of depression. The varied and overwhelming life problems confronting these patients make it difficult to distinguish realistically rooted feelings of resignation, futility and despair from more neurotically patterned reactions. On several occasions the depression seemed to be associated with the premonition of imminent demise which, at times, proved a more accurate prognostic indicator than the objective medical estimate of the facts. Is it neurotic to wish to give up the struggle when the odds are genuinely against the person involved? This is the question posed by the type of depression often experienced by stroke patients. In one way or another the depression calls attention to the real suffering associated with physical incapacity and deterioration, loneliness, abandonment and neglect (both familial and social). Not infrequently, the depressive affect is masked by stoical attitudes or simply by the absorption of the individual in habitual and automatic patterns of behavior.

The following protocols are selected to illustrate some of the varied provocative factors around which the depression becomes organized. Many of these have already been alluded to in the discussion of the life situation in which these patients find themselves.

> Case 43. 52 year old white male. Right hemiplegia. Diagnosis: Cerebral hemorrhage, left middle cerebral artery.
>
> This patient was first seen in the follow-up clinic several months after his discharge from the hospital. At that time he had recovered from what initially had been a severe aphasia, but still had a residual hemiplegia. He was unable to resume

his former occupation as a beautician and for the first time since his marriage, his wife had to become the breadwinner for the family. His prevailing mood in the home has been one of anxiety, mild depression and general irritability. The main source of these feelings seems to be the enforced inactivity of a man who previously had prided himself on his independence and enjoyment of work. He was happy, friendly and uncomplaining prior to his illness, according to the description given by his married daughter.

A not infrequent constellation of events associated with depression and bitterness occurs in the patient who, after many years of family living, finds himself alone at the time of the stroke through the loss of the mate and the lack of involvement with, or actual estrangement from the children.

> *Case 44.* 73 year old white male. Left hemiparesis. *Diagnosis:* Thrombosis, branch, right middle cerebral artery.
>
> The patient is a retired Polish-born widower. He lived with his son until two weeks prior to admission, at which time the son moved out in preparation for his imminent marriage.
>
> The patient had come to this country at the age of 21. He had worked all his life as a weaver until his retirement four years ago. His first wife died at the birth of his son. He remarried six years later. His second wife died five years ago. At one point in discussing his past life he began to cry, and said "My heart is breaking. I had a very hard life. Work, work, work. Now I get sick, terribly sick." Patient continued to express feelings of hopelessness and uselessness while in the hospital. When he felt some return of function, he began to express unrealistic notions of possibly returning to work in the same factory where his son was employed. At the end of three months he was still severely incapacitated and was discharged to a nursing home. He was again seen after he had been there three months and the depressive feelings noted during his hospital stay were still very much in evidence. He felt extremely bitter toward his son who had not been visiting him regularly.

Residual aphasic disturbances are frequently associated with depression.

> *Case 45.* Patient is a 59 year old Martinique-born French-

man. Expressive dysphasia. Paresis right arm. *Diagnosis:* Thrombosis, left middle cerebral artery.

The patient was in good health until 10 days prior to admission, when he developed some difficulty in speaking and weakness on the right side. He spoke in a monotonous, low-pitched voice, with a little slurring of the consonants. He had difficulty in naming about a third of the objects presented to him. He tired readily, at which time his speech difficulty became more manifest. When seen several weeks after admission, his speech had improved, but the combination of his accent and the residual dysphasia made communication difficult. He also tended to speak in a very low, barely audible voice. He cried frequently in the course of the interview. He became obviously disturbed when he encountered difficulty in self-expression and perseveration was apt to occur. His affect was that of resignation and depression, and at one point he said he no longer cared what happened to him.

He appeared considerably improved when seen six months after discharge, despite the fact that he still had a residual expressive speech deficit. Depressive moods tended to recur, but generally lasted only a short time. He did not cry as often as formerly. The crying, when it did occur, was usually precipitated by the difficulty he still had in maintaining an even flow of conversation.

In the next two patients more severe and enduring depressive reactions occurred. In the first instance it was associated with visual complaints initially and then with blindness which became complete following a second stroke two and a half years later. This was followed by gradual physical deterioration and death. In both instances the depression seemed to presage dire consequences.

Case 46. 65 year old white female. Left hemianopia. *Diagnosis:* Thrombosis, right middle cerebral artery.

This patient was first seen eleven months after her discharge from the hospital. At that time her chief complaint was inability to see other than vague outlines and shadows. The only objective finding on neurological examination was a residual left hemianopia.

The patient was born in Poland and had been in this

country for 43 years. She was married for 45 years and had
three married children. Her husband worked as a waiter until
his retirement. He described a striking change in his wife's behavior and appearance since the occurrence of the stroke. She
had been an energetic, enterprising and capable person. There
had been no depressive episodes. The picture he painted now
was one of a gradually deepening depression. She refused to
get about by herself in the home and had become completely
dependent upon her husband. He, in turn, was fearful of
leaving her alone because of her frequent mention of suicide
and his discovery on one occasion that she had left the gas
jets on.

The patient described the change in herself as follows:

"There is some difference. Before, I dressed different. I went
among people. I sit on the couch the whole day now. I can't
do much on the couch. The eyes are the main thing. Everybody gets up in the morning and has light. I sit in darkness.
Can the doctor give me back the life I had before?"

All social life had ceased and there was very little contact
with any of the children. The husband was forced to take over
all of the household responsibilities. The patient's premorbid
personality, as seen through the eyes of her daughter, was that
of a rather cold and undemonstrative person who never seemed
very deeply or genuinely concerned with her children. Although
the mother was superficially friendly and active in many chari-
table and social organizations, the daughter feels she had no
close friends. The daughter obviously found it easier to understand her mother's present self-concern and dependency than
the husband did.

Repeated efforts were made to convince the husband of the
need for psychiatric hospitalization. Although he was willing,
he yielded to her entreaties about not being separated from
him. When such hospitalization was finally brought about,
he signed her out when she refused to submit to shock treatment.

A second stroke occurred 2½ years after the first. It was
ushered in by a period of initial confusion and the loss of her
remaining vision. It is of interest that almost immediately the
depression lifted. This was noted both in the tone and vigor
of her speech and her verbalization:

"I feel a little freer. I feel everything will be all right. I don't feel so much depressed. I want to go home to my husband and children. The doctors should do for me what is possible (in contrast to her earlier implied insistence that something be done to restore her vision)."

When the patient was seen four months following her discharge, the clinical picture had reverted back to one of chronic depression and helpless dependency.

Case 47.   83 year old white male. Transitory left hemiparesis. Diagnosis: Thrombosis, right middle cerebral artery.

When first seen, the patient was alert, responsive, eager for contact and looked and acted younger than his age. He was born in Hungary and came to this country alone at the age of 16. The quality of his existence is best expressed in his own words:

"I came here alone at the age of 16 and I went to school to learn English. They started me off in a cigar-making factory. I didn't work there long, maybe three or four years, and then I said to myself, 'This isn't the life.' They paid me poorly. There was no future and my family didn't help me out. They were poor and ignorant. I was very good at that work. A big concern gave me a job. They taught me how to be a foreman. I worked there over ten years. The girls looked up to me. I was a nice-looking fellow and young. I liked to keep company with girls but not to get married. I didn't make enough money. My ambition was to settle down on a solid foundation. So I didn't really live. I didn't want to get married like an ignorant fool. When I needed a woman I paid her and then good-bye."

He spoke of his retirement ten years earlier with regret. "I don't like it. I can't bring back the young years. I look for a job and they laugh at me because of my age."

He described his reaction to his illness: "I didn't think I was going to get sick like this. I can't walk. I can't use my arm. I'd like to go home, go to sleep and never wake up. I don't mean I would ever kill myself. I've just over-leased my time."

The hemiparesis cleared in the course of the next two months except for some residual weakness in the left upper extremity. Despite this, there was a general deterioration in his physical condition. He presented multiple somatic complaints, some of which, on investigation, proved referable to osteoarthritis of the cervical spine and poor peripheral circulation in both lower extremities. He ate and slept poorly. He was transferred to the Rehabilitation Service but felt too weak to participate in any organized program of activity. He became increasingly depressed and voiced his dissatisfaction with himself, his surroundings and the ward personnel. He began to lose hope of ever leaving the hospital when a brother upon whom he was counting to arrange for his care left the city. He refused to consider a nursing home or any other placement. He gradually became completely bedridden and died seven months after his admission to the hospital. Autopsy revealed severe generalized arteriosclerotic changes.

Comment: At the time the stroke occurred the patient's existence was in a state of precarious balance both physically and emotionally. From the physical point of view, the causative factors accounting for his death existed for many years before the stroke, to the point where the degree of reserve in his vital organs was almost depleted. From the psychological point of view, his relatedness to his surroundings had grown very tenuous and his sense of usefulness to himself and to others had been considerably undermined since his retirement. The stroke was, in effect, an incidental occurrence which simply served to expose and accentuate the underlying deteriorating processes at work. At some point there was an intuitive realization by the patient that this was the case. The struggle to live was renounced and the depression came into the picture as an effort by the patient to justify his decision to cooperate in the process of dying.

CHAPTER V

PSYCHIATRIC HOSPITALIZATION

The need for the psychiatric hospitalization of stroke patients arises in the following circumstances in this order of frequency:

(1) A degree of organic dementia resulting in behavioral deficits too difficult to manage in a medical ward or nursing home.

(2) Depressive reactions to severe aphasia without significant intellectual deterioration.

(3) Episodic, uncontrollable outbreaks, generally with assaultive, obscene or negativistic behavior.

(4) The late occurrence of psychiatric manifestations following repeated failure to adapt to the altered life situation imposed by the residual deficits.

(5) The apparent precipitation by the stroke of a latent psychotic process, the degree of brain damage playing a relatively unimportant role.

1. ORGANIC DEMENTIA

Case 48. 85 year old white female. Disorientation, confusion, left hemiplegia. *Diagnosis:* Thrombosis, right middle cerebral-internal carotid system.

The patient was unmindful of the examiner's presence. From time to time she would call out in a loud and raucous voice "I want to make a wee-wee." At other times she interjected remarks out of context such as "I love everybody," or "Dorothy, make coffee." She did not respond to direct questioning except to give her name. On occasion, if she were aroused sufficiently, she was able to give a pertinent answer. In this manner it was learned that she was widowed for 30 years and has three children. Her attention would then drift away from the examiner and she would again verbalize her preoccupation with her urinary urge. Once she was able to name the year correctly but did not know the month.

2. REACTIVE DEPRESSION ASSOCIATED WITH SEVERE EXPRESSIVE APHASIA

Case 49. 69 year old white male. Gradual onset of right hemiparesis. Expressive aphasia following angiography. *Diagnosis:* Thrombosis, left internal carotid artery.

The patient had been admitted to the hospital with a history of progressive weakness of the right arm and leg of four months' duration. Arteriography was performed to rule out an expanding lesion. Expressive aphasia set in immediately following the operation. The patient was under observation on the ward for a period of three months following the acute onset of the almost total expressive aphasia. By the end of that time there was a limited improvement in speech. He had difficulty naming the hospital. He was unable to state his home address, becoming confused when he attempted to articulate the numbers involved. He was able to communicate sufficiently for some historical data to be obtained. The patient was born in Russia and had been in this country for 45 years. He worked as a tailor until his retirement four years ago. He was married at the age of 36 but separated after only three weeks. He drank moderately but never had delirium tremens. His siblings remained in Russia and he had no family in this country.

Following the occurrence of the aphasia he became increasingly morose and withdrawn. At times it was reported that he was out of contact and experiencing hallucinatory episodes. When questioned about this, no history of auditory or visual hallucinations could be elicited. The patient did admit to experiencing acute anxiety at night and having frequent nightmares. The depression gradually deepened, centering mainly around what he felt was the lack of any further improvement in his speech. He was transferred at the end of three months to the psychiatric service because of the likelihood of a suicidal attempt.

3. RESISTIVE NEGATIVISTIC BEHAVIOR

Case 50. 65 year old white male. Right hemiparesis. *Diagnosis:* Thrombosis, left middle cerebral-internal carotid system.

The patient was admitted to the hospital following the sudden onset of weakness of the right side and loss of consciousness. He had had a previous stroke a year and a half before, with a transitory aphasia and a mild residual right hemiparesis. At the time of the present admission he was generally negativistic and resistive and showed no spontaneous speech. During the first two weeks he lay in bed with either a vacant or glaring expression on his face. He appeared to refuse rather than to be unable to engage in verbal communication. At the end of three weeks he appeared more responsive. His answers tended to be very abbreviated and approximate and were more accurate concerning earlier personal history than current orientation. However, there was no spontaneous participation in the interpersonal situation and he quickly lapsed into a withdrawn silence unless persistent efforts were made to engage his attention.

The following exchange was characteristic:

Q. What is the name of this place?
A. Bellevue.
Q. Where is it?
A. Right outside.
Q. How did you get here?
A. I was picked up.
Q. What was the matter?
A. I couldn't tell you.
Q. Did anything happen to you?
A. I couldn't tell you.
Q. What is the date?
A. The 8th. (Actually November 5, 1958.)
Q. Of what?
A. I couldn't tell you.
Q. What year is this?
A. I couldn't tell you.
Q. What is your address?
A. 280. (Incorrect.)
Q. How old are you?
A. I don't know.
Q. What kind of work do you do?
A. Machinist. (True.)

The negativistic, oppositional behavior recurred episodically and three weeks after admission psychiatric transfer was necessary when the patient made repeated efforts to leave the hospital in his pajamas.

4. UNCONTROLLABLE ASSAULTIVE BEHAVIOR AS A LATE SEQUEL

Case 51. Patient is a 34 year old white male. Right hemiparesis. Severe expressive aphasia. *Diagnosis:* Embolus, left middle cerebral artery.

The patient was first seen a year after the onset of the stroke. The onset occurred suddenly with unconsciousness, right hemiplegia and loss of speech. Confusion persisted over a two-week period.

The patient was born in Poland of a peasant family. He had approximately four years of schooling and then left home to be on his own. During the war he managed to get to England, where he joined the Polish Army. He met his wife there and they were married in 1948. She was eight years his senior and had a son by an earlier marriage. Their own son was born in England. They emigrated to this country in 1951. He has since been employed as a window cleaner.

From the wife's description the patient appears to have been a taciturn, irritable, somewhat withdrawn individual. Compliant to authority outside the home, he was often bossy and abusive in the home. He has been unable to work since his illness and spends most of his time in idleness about the house. He was impatient and irritable with the child and very demanding with his wife.

His speech remained limited to a few fragmented automatisms. He was able to communicate more effectively through writing. He seemed to minimize or even deny his speech difficulty. He persisted in attempts to participate in the conversation despite the repeated occurrence of great impatience and annoyance when he was unable to do so.

In the course of the subsequent year the deterioration at home became noticeably worse. Repeated efforts at job placement failed. There was no further return of speech. The stepson, with whom the patient never did get along, returned from the army to live at home. This constellation of events resulted in more frequent and more violent abusive outbursts toward his wife. She finally accepted psychiatric hospitalization for her husband when during one episode he went after her with a large kitchen knife.

5. THE APPEARANCE OF OVERT PSYCHOTIC SYMPTOMS FOLLOWING A STROKE

Case 52. The patient is a 72 year old white male. Right hemiparesis. *Diagnosis:* Thrombosis, left middle cerebral artery.

The patient was admitted to the hospital for gastro-intestinal bleeding. The gradual onset of weakness in the right arm and leg was noted two weeks after admission. History from the family indicated some emotional lability over the past year manifest mainly in the tendency to cry. He was described as an eccentric and isolated individual who began to withdraw from social contacts in the year preceding his illness. He saw little of his relatives and shared nothing of his life with them. He had come to this country from Bulgaria and had worked as a blacksmith until four or five years ago. He was never married and has always lived alone. He spoke quite readily in the following vein about himself: "I'm dealing with God. He gives me all kinds of information. I have four books and each book is filled up with what God told me and with what God showed me. It's like a dream. Moses, Jesus, Mohammed, all saw God while dreaming. I see what He shows me. I figure there will be a big revolution, a big exchange in the world. Before I came to this country I was shown many different things by God."

He seemed completely unperturbed by the paradox of his exalted state on the one hand and his actual state of illness and dependency on the other. Despite the preoccupation with his delusional system, he was able to respond appropriately to the demands of the ward situation. Psychiatric hospitalization was effected after his bleeding duodenal ulcer had been controlled.

Comment: The patient presented a lifelong history of a deviant and schizoid personality pattern. It is also apparent that some degree of psychological decompensation had set in for at least a year before the stroke occurred. What occurred after the stroke was simply a more unabashed public presentation of his delusional preoccupations.

CHAPTER VI

THE REHABILITATION PROCESS AND STROKE PATIENTS

Some of the general aspects of the problems met with in the rehabilitation process of stroke patients can be inferred from the foregoing clinical material. In this study only patients with a residual motor deficit were selected for an active rehabilitation program, and patients with serious medical complications or serious impairment in mental functioning were excluded. Aphasia itself, in the absence of intellectual deterioration, was not considered a contraindication. The selective process thus eliminated that segment of the stroke population which got well spontaneously and those patients whose mental changes were severe enough to prevent effective participation in a rehabilitation program.

The central theoretical difficulty which arises in connection with the task of evaluating the progress of these patients centers about the concept of motivation. What is good motivation? How is motivation related to the capacity of the individual? How do pre-existing personality difficulties emerge in the rehabilitation setting and what role do they play in limiting the recovery potential of the patient?

Whenever a patient fails to achieve the estimated potential of functional recovery, any of three evaluations may be made of the situation:

1. The patient does not want to get better.

2. The patient unconsciously strives to limit his own movement toward recovery.

3. The patient does not have the capacity to get better, that is, the estimate was wrong.

Category 1 may theoretically apply in the case of depressed

patients who at a conscious level renounce the struggle to get well. Where such renunciation is total and complete (as in Case 47) it is more apt to be a reflection of an inability to participate in the program rather than a desire not to.

If Category 3 obtains, the original estimate made by the observer has to be revised. An estimate made purely on the degree of motor loss may now have to take into account difficulties stemming from what Kurt Goldstein refers to as impairment of the "abstract attitude." Difficulties of this order include limited attention span, distractibility, poor retention, difficulty in initiating new tasks, and the tendency to cling to patterns of more familiar behavior. With patients of this type profound reactions to failure occur and the intensity and meaning of these reactions for the patient must be appreciated. The task set before the patient must be limited to one new item at a time. When the environmental field provides more stimuli than the patient can effectively master, especially when the patient is being led into areas of new activity, the so-called "catastrophic reaction" is apt to occur. Intense anxiety, disorganized behavior and fear of the task at hand result. The same intense reaction occurs if the factor of ready fatigability is overlooked.

Very few patients actually fall into category 2. Neurotic mechanisms oriented toward secondary gain occurred occasionally in a few inadequate individuals who had established an institutional way of life and sought to maintain it. More characteristic were those patients who strove hard to recover some functional use of the impaired extremities and who vigorously sought to reestablish an independent way of life. If anything impaired the rehabilitation process it was more apt to be the excessive zeal, impatience and overestimation of feasible goals by the patient. The following example is an illustration of this type of reaction in extreme measure.

Case 53.   73 year old white male. Right hemiplegia. Aphasia. *Diagnosis:* Thrombosis, branch, left middle cerebral artery.

The onset occurred with loss of consciousness and for the first two weeks in the hospital the patient was in poor contact. A tracheotomy was necessary soon after admission. There was a gradual improvement and he was discharged after two months.

Speech had returned but there was a residual right hemiparesis. He was readmitted five months later with a second stroke on the same side. Speech was difficult to understand and he appeared depressed. He complained about the rehabilitation service, saying that they would not let him use a cane. Actually, the rehabilitation personnel found him very uncooperative and stubborn. He refused to accept the fact that he was not ready for a cane, despite the fact that on several occasions when he was given a cane he came close to falling. He had his own ideas of what was best for him and was unable to accept any compromise.

Another type of unconscious mechanism impeding effective progress in rehabilitation is that of denial. In one patient (Case 24) the unrealistic attitude toward illness led her to eschew the use of a cane as a symbol of being crippled. She would attempt to walk about either by leaning against a wall or by unobtrusively pushing a chair in front of her. She had from the very inception of her illness shown a consistent pattern of denying the reality of her illness. Initially the pattern took a delusional form with the insistence that the paralyzed arm did not belong to her, but was the arm of her dead husband. The delusional elements disappeared, but the tendency to avoid facing the real implications of her handicap persisted throughout the three-year period of observation. The use of the cane was a tacit admission of a handicap she was not prepared to accept.

The key to the understanding of the problem of motivation lies in not separating the problem of motivation from the problem of capacity. What determines whether a person is motivated to a certain act is in part whether or not he can perform the act successfully and in part what his concept of the implications of such a performance are for his total life situation. The normal individual strives to enhance his capacity for the performance of such acts that he anticipates will enhance his life situation. The brain-damaged patient is juggling the same set of equations but with different elements entering the picture. Success or failure occurs in an all-or-none fashion for him rather than as a gradient with a potential for growth through trial and error. It is the immediate result which counts rather than the fruits of a long-sustained effort. Mastery and motivation become much more closely interwoven. When a patient (cf. Case 40) fumes and rants at the incompetency of the various members of the rehabilitation team and vents his anger at everyone connected with the hospital for not getting him back on his feet, he is in the first place setting excessively high goals for himself in the rehabilitation process and then expressing self-rage and intolerance of the helplessness and anxiety precipitated by his failure to master the tasks and achieve his goal. In this instance only a lowering of the expectations of the patient can make for a more efficient participation in the program. This is in contrast to patients in the third category, where the reverse holds true. In the latter, the program set by the staff has to be tailored to meet the capacity of the patient.

Any concern with the problem of motivation therefore leads directly into the question of what is the capacity of the patient in respect to a given task set by the environment and what are the factors limiting this capacity. These in turn may be primarily psychological insofar as they relate essentially to the personality pattern and aspirations, or secondarily psychological if they basically reflect limitations imposed by the altered brain milieu. In the first instance, the therapeutic approach is oriented primarily toward bringing about a change in the individual. In the second instance the utmost flexibility has to be achieved in the patterning of the environmental stimuli so as to prevent any situation from occurring where too great a distance develops between the skills, confidence and courage required by certain tasks and the patient's capacity to provide these ingredients.

CHAPTER VII

DIRECTIONAL CHANGES

In most instances the occurrence of the stroke is realistically integrated into the prevailing life pattern. It is only in the exceptional case that there occurs a sharp alteration in the general direction of the patient's life attributable to defects in motivation rather than physical deficit. The patients who falter and swerve in their direction are not necessarily the sickest from a psychiatric point of view. A number of schizophrenics in the study integrated their experience in a way which enabled them to continue their previous schizophrenic mode of adaptation in the same compensated and stabilized manner (Case 36). On the other hand, many patients who underwent profound personality changes following the stroke appeared to have functioned in a stable manner throughout most of their lives.

What this points up is the need to focus not on an abstract appraisal of psychopathological patterns but on understanding the current life situation and the consequent meaning of the stroke to the patient at this particular moment in his life. Repeatedly one gets the feeling in talking with these patients that had the stroke occurred a year or two earlier or a year or two later, their reactions would have been quite different. At times it climaxes a process of resignation and surrender set in motion years before; at other times it initiates such a process. In some patients it touches off a last-ditch stand dedicated to the pursuit of unattained life goals and ambitions. Occasionally it opens up new vistas for the elaboration of secondary gain from illness. Unrealistic strivings for independence and unrealistic dependency are perhaps the two main channels into which irrational modes of adaptation flow.

Major directional changes follow from the nature and severity of the residual deficits and take the form generally of (a) inability to continue to be gainfully employed; (b) dependency within the home situation with the loss of the usual sources of social and personal satisfactions; (c) nursing home placement, and finally in some instances (d) psychiatric hospitalization. The impact of some of these changes has been mentioned in connection with several of the patients presented. These are the gross adjustments to living foisted on the patient by the illness. When the patients who were able to return home were followed in the clinic for a period of two years, a number of interesting fine adjustments were observed.

Four patients who had a history of heavy drinking prior to the stroke stopped completely after their illness. In the case of two of these patients, the main factor appeared to be the residual physical deficit which prevented the patient from getting about as freely as formerly, in one instance because of general weakness, and in one because of an expressive aphasia.

In two other patients, however, the renunciation of their dependency upon alcohol was part of their orientation towards a more constructive way of life. Both were in the younger age group.

The first was a 41 year old white female (Case 22) with a residual mild left hemiparesis following a cerebral embolus. Prior to the onset of her stroke this patient had frequent bouts of illness directly or indirectly related to an underlying rheumatic condition. Despite this she struggled very hard to take care of her family consisting of her husband and three children, ranging in age from ten to nineteen. In addition she held down a part-time job. She was chronically depressed and drank up to a pint of whiskey a day. A few years ago she attempted suicide by turning the gas jets on. The stroke brought about two significant changes in her life. In the first place, it made her physically incapable of carrying anywhere near the workload she formerly had. Secondly, and perhaps more important, it brought home to her the sudden realization of how exploited she had been by other members of her family.

"I realized now I have to fight to stay alive. Before, they all took me for granted. 'Why isn't this done? Why isn't that done?' He (the husband) was like a big child. He thought he was the only one in the family. I decided to sit down and talk it over with him. He was not to leave everything up to me. Now he knows I can't do it and that's all."

This reversal after 24 years of married life had repercussions in other areas. She reported that her husband had become more affectionate and that their sexual life had improved.

Case 54. 45 year old Negro male. *Diagnosis:* Subarachnoid hemorrhage secondary to ruptured aneurysm.

This patient drank heavily for many years and had several hospitalizations for alcoholism. He denied ever having delirium tremens. He has lived with three different women over extended periods of time, resulting in a total of seven illegitimate children, the oldest of whom is 27. He was arrested once for non-support. He spent three years in the Army and apparently had a good record. He was unperturbed by his recent illness and seemed eager to leave the hospital. Although his mode of life had become somewhat stabilized in recent years, there were residual sources of instability associated with his drinking and his tendency to flee from responsibility and to uproot himself when his burdens became too difficult.

Over the course of a year and a half following his discharge from the hospital there was a remarkable transformation in this patient. He became more settled, serious and insightful. Concerning the fact that he was no longer drinking or carousing, he remarked: "If it means a lot to your health, you've got to give it up." He seems more genuinely concerned with his family responsibilities. He has been working on and off as a laborer and turning his earnings over to his wife.

Patients react differently to the enduring state of invalidism and dependency ushered in by the stroke. In the next patient there was an acceptance of the dependency as a kind of interim situation of indefinite duration before more complete recovery occurred and a deep conviction that such recovery would occur.

Case 55. 50 year old white male. Pseudo-bulbar palsy. *Diagnosis:* Thrombosis, basilar artery.

The stroke occurred in June, 1958. The patient was severely ill initially. A tracheotomy was necessary at the time of admission. For several months he was confined to a wheel chair and was unable to speak because of a marked dysarthria. After the acute phase had subsided the patient responded eagerly to the program of exercises and physiotherapy. His affective responses were always positively tinged, even when he was almost completely helpless. There was a forced, over-reactive quality to his responses, but always in the direction of expressing optimism, cheerfulness and confidence.

The patient was born in this country, and had worked most of his life as a shipping clerk. He was married but had separated from his wife over twenty years before. He appeared to be of dull normal intelligence and was content to lead a very circumscribed life. His interests were limited to watching television and following sports. He has not seen his child, who is now over 20, since his separation. He has a sister who relates to him in a maternal kind of fashion.

His response to the first year in the nursing home was as follows: "I get along very nice. Only trouble is that I cough when I drink fluids. The nursing home isn't too bad, only there isn't enough therapy. I do my own exercise. I don't want anyone to know where I am. There are too many old people here."

Comment: This patient's illness, despite its stormy course, precipitated him into a milieu in which he was the object of considerable personal attention and interest and one in which his own strivings toward recovery met with a warm and appreciative audience. He responded with a kind of childlike basking in the approbation of those who were working with him. Despite his residual physical incapacities, his life was perhaps less circumscribed than it had been before because of the new social elements introduced, first in the hospital and later in the nursing home and the continued relationships associated with the follow-up clinic.

In another patient (Case 46), there was the not infrequent paradoxical occurrence of a gradual deepening of the dependency along with vociferous protestations to the effect that this was an unwanted and offensive form of existence. Guilt and defensiveness seem to be an inevitable accompaniment of the dependent state. In lesser measure this was also true of another patient (Case 43). His verbalization centered mainly about the feelings of self-disgust and loss of self-esteem associated with his physical incapacity, and the necessity of his wife's working. When the daughter was interviewed, another side of the picture came into focus. The patient had grown more and more demanding and was gradually relinquishing many activities he was capable of doing. The toll that this kind of reaction takes on the other person, the wife in this instance, is considerable. What is also apparent in cases like the two above is that whatever the cost, the relationship appeared to be indissoluble. In others, however, particularly in younger people, the reaction of the mate and the possibility of rejection and desertion pose additional problems.

Case 56. 31 year old Negro male. Left hemiplegia. *Diagnosis:* Subarachnoid hemorrhage secondary to ruptured aneurysm.

This patient was left with a severe residual hemiplegia. Prior to his illness he had been a parking lot attendant. He has been married for 17 years and has two children, ages 16 and 13. He was born in Charleston, S. C. He left school in the sixth grade to take on odd jobs. He had gonorrhea at the age of 15 and had been arrested on two occasions, once for fighting and once following an auto accident. He appeared to be a good-natured, easy-going and somewhat lethargic type of person. There was some naiveté and lack of concern both about the illness and his own future. He seemed to take it for granted that he would get well and would be accepted back on his old job. Pulmonary tuberculosis was diagnosed during his hospital stay and he remained in a tuberculosis hospital for almost a year following his discharge. When he was again seen a year and a half after the onset of his illness he was spending most of his time at home in idleness. His wife was working. His oldest child had to leave school and go to work. In the course of the next year his relationship with his wife began to deteriorate rapidly. He kept putting off making any serious effort to seek help in regard to possible employment and did nothing along these lines until his wife insisted that he leave. She made it clear that she was tired of supporting him and wished to end the relationship. They had had no physical relations for the past six months and each had gone their own way in fulfilling their needs. When last seen their break-up appeared imminent.

The problem of social stigmatization sometimes figures prominently in the reactions of younger patients.

Case 57. 43 year old Negro female. Left hemiplegia. *Diagnosis:* Aneurysm, right internal carotid artery.

Prior to her illness this patient had been a cafeteria worker. Her first common-law marriage occurred in 1933. They separated in 1941. "I've had bad luck with men. Other women take them away." She had been living with another man since 1947. "He's giving me a hard time. He's had another woman since 1956. He wants me to get on my high heel shoes and get running just like his other girl friend." She expressed considerable bitterness towards her husband. She is chronically depressed, cries easily, and has occasional thoughts of suicide. Her mistrustfulness of her husband extends to other people. She regards them as "nosey." They ask too many questions. "People talk so much. They probably think it's a stroke. I don't know what to tell them. I tell them it's a shock. They make a person depressed. It's embarrassing when they see me with a stick. They're very nosey around my way. They mind everybody's business."

CHAPTER VIII

SEXUAL SEQUELAE

The sexual interests and activities of people in their seventh, eighth or even ninth decade are enormously varied so that the individual differences noted in our stroke population for the most part simply reflect the general trends in this age population. One woman of 69, when asked if she had physical relations with her husband, replied: "Sure we do. What do you think? Of course we sleep together." Occasionally, however, when there is a sharp change in the pattern of sexual activity, the relationship to the occurrence of the stroke is quite clear.

The most frequent change following the stroke is the occurrence of impotence in the face of continuing desire. The repercussions of this may be minimal or highly distressing, depending upon the patient's age and life situation. In one patient (Case 5) the impotence was accepted as an incidental and not too important after-effect of illness. He was a 65 year old Turkish male who had been separated from his wife for the past eight years. Since that time he had been having sexual relations three or four times a month with various women friends of his. He described the situation as follows: "I was very passionate before. Since I left the hospital up to now (a year later) it's been dead. It's too soft. Now it's just like my hand (referring to the residual paralysis of his left arm)—dead. Sometimes I have an orgasm and it's soft." The patient spoke about these changes with some regret, but without too much concern. He expressed real distress at his estrangement from his daughter, whom he feels his wife turned against him.

In another and younger patient (Case 19), the same symptom resulted in considerable distress. He was 57 and first seen at the time of his second stroke. He was married and had a son of 23.

He had been a restaurant worker most of his life. Although he succeeded in carrying out most of the activities of daily living, his second stroke did leave him home-bound. Most of his time was spent sitting before a television set. He spontaneously reported that since his last illness he had been unable to have an erection. He experienced sexual feeling but remained impotent. Prior to this last episode he had been having intercourse with his wife twice weekly. His sexual handicap, as well as the occurrence of the second stroke itself, resulted in an anxious and depressed reaction which he was struggling to control.

Sometimes one suspects there is a difficulty in this area which the patient appears to evade or deny. When one patient, age 44, was questioned about his feelings two and a half months following the onset of the stroke, he denied having any desire at the present time, but hastened to add: "I've got plenty of time for that. I'm not a hog. You can take your time for that."

Sexual references during the early phase of the illness, especially when associated with confusional states, are not at all uncommon. This was noted in two patients previously considered. A 75 year old white woman (Case 39) began making veiled references to sexual activities going on about her on the ward, especially by the Negro attendants. Another patient (Case 24) experienced a succession of sexually tinged responses, each successive response becoming less specific and more impersonal. When seen soon after admission she insisted that the paralyzed arm (left) was that of her dead husband and that she had awakened during the night to find it resting on her breast with the feeling that he was caressing her. The next day she no longer attributed the arm to her husband, but insisted that he was still in the hospital and lying in the bed next to her. This response disappeared in the course of the next two weeks, and at the same time that it did the sexual theme emerged in a different guise. Opposite her on the ward was a patient who had had a craniotomy and whose hair at the time had just begun to grow back. The patient misidentified her as a male, accused the nurses of smuggling a man into the ward, lifting the covers from his bed and playing with him.

These changes, as Weinstein and Kahn have shown (4), are

not direct manifestations of changes in the sexual sphere secondary to the stroke, but indicate rather that these patients are expressing in sexual terms whatever current conflict is uppermost in their lives. This altered mode of self-expression relates primarily to the existence of diffuse alterations in brain milieu and not to any real change in sexual functioning. Such was the case with both of the patients (Cases 39 and 24) referred to above. In the first the central conflict had to do with the sense of sudden upheaval, the feeling of helplessness and incarceration, and the fear of being at the mercy of people for whom in the past she had contempt. In the second patient the sexual references expressed in experiential terms how she felt about her own paralyzed arm, namely, the fact that it felt dead, separate from her, and that when it rested on a sensitive part of her body it felt like a caress externally administered. Her delusion or illusion about the nurses manipulating the helpless "male" patient was a further reflection of her own feelings following the manipulation of the paralyzed arm and the incidental sexual responses elicited when it rested on her breast.

CHAPTER IX

ANOSOGNOSIA AND RELATED DISORDERS

The occurrence of a sudden diffuse alteration in brain milieu—a situation that characterizes the moderately to severely ill stroke patient—is often associated with unawareness of illness, unawareness of defect, and, in some instances, unawareness of the defective part itself. The term anosognosia was originally introduced by Babinski (5) to denote the unawareness of a hemiplegia following a vascular accident. It is now more generally used to refer to unawareness of any aspect of a disease process when this is associated with brain damage. These manifestations have been variously interpreted and there is as yet no general agreement concerning their etiology and significance. It has remained, however, an area holding much interest both for the neurologist and the psychiatrist. Critchley, in a recent contribution, sums up the current diversity of opinion concerning the nature of anosognosia and offers a constructive comment:

"There has been no complete unanimity among neurologists concerning the nature or causation of anosognosia. Briefly, there are three chief opinions about the matter: (1) That anosognosia is a specific 'parietal' syndrome; furthermore, that it is the expression of the minor hemisphere; and that the minor (nondominant) parietal lobe is more concerned with the integrity of corporeal awareness (body-image) than is the dominant half of the brain. (2) That the all-important factor is not so much the *site* of the lesion, or even the *side* of the lesion, as the degree of accompanying confusion and the nature of the previous personality. (3) That anosognosia for hemiplegia is merely the most striking and the most easily recognizable instance of what is indeed a common and even characteristic feature of cerebral disease in general, namely, a failure to realize or admit the presence or extent of disability resulting therefrom. In other words, anosognosia is but one example of the ordinary 'denial syndrome' of a neurological patient. These three conceptions constitute the main uncertainties which surround the topic.

"Although the three hypotheses mentioned are often discussed as though they were mutually exclusive, this is not necessarily true. In other words, it may be a fact that anosognosia for hemiplegia is more often seen with lesions of the parietal lobe than with lesions elsewhere in the brain—though clinical exceptions may perhaps occur. Secondly, a certain type of personality existing before the hemiplegia may well play some part in determining the patient's subsequent attitude toward his disability. Thirdly, it may well be that anosognosia for hemiplegia cannot exist with a perfectly clear sensorium. Fourthly, anosognosia can also follow lesions of the dominant half of the brain, through less readily identifiable" (6, p. 285).

Critchley's categories may be further reduced to two main theoretical orientations, one tending toward the concept of a specific and localizable defect and the other toward a holistic and organismic approach. In the monograph containing their own views, Weinstein and Kahn (4) present an excellent historical review of the leading exponents of both points of view. Among those who have regarded anosognosia as a unitary and localizable defect, many have regarded it as peculiar to lesions of the minor parietal lobe (7 and 8).

The most recent contribution based on the concept of a specific type of deficit is that of Denny-Brown and his associates (9). They have advanced the concept of amorphosynthesis or defective spatial summation of stimuli. This occurs contralaterally to either damaged parietal lobe in contrast to aphasic defects or disorders involving the perception of symbols. The latter are almost always the result of damage to the dominant hemisphere and the resulting difficulties involve both sides of extra-personal space. In the case of amorphosynthesis, there is no defect in the reception of any of the primary sensations. The symptoms result from the defective perception of the spatial aspects of all forms of sensations arising in the opposite side of the body. Associated with this is a greater vulnerability of such perceptions in rivalry with more clearly differentiated stimuli from the sound side. It is in this way that the phenomena of extinction are related to defective spatial summation. There is poor differentiation of the extinguished stimulus in competition with the more highly differentiated stimulus.

Extending this hypothesis, the authors account for the phenomenon of anosognosia. The perception of the existence of a limb or the disability of it can suffer extinction if the spatial disorder is sufficiently extensive and if the normal side provides highly differentiated sensation of its presence. This effect can be produced by both right and left parieto-occipital lesions. In each case there may result a lack of recognition of the opposite half of the body and the opposite half of extra-personal space (imperception of the body, spatial inattention).

Two types of phenomena may be recognized in connection with this deficit. Anosognosia and related effects such as apraxia of dressing represent the severest degree of loss of that part of parietal function having to do with bodily sensation. Visual inattention and related disorders such as defective copying, distortion of visual coordinates, errors in visuo-spatial judgment, loss of spatial localization and denial of blindness represent varying degrees of impairment of the visual component of parietal function. Amorphosynthesis may thus be regarded as a disturbance in cortical function manifest as a disturbance in behavior. It is important to differentiate the effects directly related to this deficit and the attitude of the patient toward his symptoms and the verbal account he may give of what he perceives. Secondary factors are introduced which are rooted in the personality of the patient.

In short, the point of view expressed by these observers is that anosognosia is the result of ineffective sensory synthesis by the parietal lobe with consequent loss of cortical stimulus value from the opposite sensory fields in the motivation of behavior. It represents "a mental aversion rather than a repression, a mental 'avoiding response' comparable to the motor reaction of the hand and allied to the peculiar retracting avoiding reactions we have found in monkeys with parietal lesions" (10, p. 32).

The objections[1] raised to this, as well as any other point of view based on a unitary modality of dysfunction, are threefold: 1) Extensive parietal lobe impairment may occur without this phenomenon being present.   2) Extensive denial may occur with relatively minor sensory impairment.   3) The effects of diffuse brain damage are minimized or overlooked.

Weinstein and Kahn approach the problem of anosognosia and denial in an entirely different way. They regard these manifestations as modes of adaptation to stress rather than as individual defects. They emphasize the fact that some motivation to deny illness exists in everyone. The significant difference between the normal and the brain-damaged patient is that in the latter alterations occur in the perceptual-symbolic organization of the language in which the denial is expressed. In a milieu of diffuse brain dysfunction anything may be denied that the patient feels is wrong with him. Patients with explicit verbal denial of illness tend to ignore and rationalize illness and to deny felt inadequacies which existed before the brain damage occurred.

Central to Weinstein and Kahn's interpretation is their concept of language not as labels but as the product of a pattern of interaction between the individual and his environment. "In language we not only classify the environment but express a relatedness in it from which we derive a sense of reality. . ." (11, pp. 964-965). "The feeling of the reality of one's experience is related to the degree to which the symbolic representation identifies one with the values of his culture" (11, p. 965). In the language of denial motivational factors are expressed in terms of selected aspects of the environment. The latter may be classified into spatial, temporal, personal and somatic aspects. Disorientation and reduplication, for example, represent the reorganization of the spatial and temporal aspects of the environment expressing the prevailing motivation of the patient under conditions of altered brain milieu. Confabulation represents an interaction with the temporal aspect of the environment in terms of altering the temporal sequence of events.

---

[1] Cf. Weinstein and Kahn, ref. No. 4.

It is this altered pattern of symbolic expression rather than the particular elements themselves which is related to the level of brain dysfunction. The "language" of denial includes, in addition to explicit verbal denial, such effects as disorientation, reduplication, and paraphasia. The last-mentioned term as defined by Weinstein and Kahn is an altered mode of interaction in terms of misnaming objects. The misnamed object is related to the patient's problem. A single aspect of the structure or function of the object emerges in the distortion. Other manifestations include the occurrence of the withdrawn, akinetic state and altered sexual behavior. These are not to be regarded as individual defects that can be represented in anatomical or physiological terms, but are examples of differences in the level of integration of language. They are related to features in the premorbid personality rather than to differently situated cortical lesions. The alterations in language provide a means of identification with such aspects of the cultural environment as health, illness, home and work, violence and death. One's feeling of reality is more related to one's relationship to his environment than to any more logical thought process. To be ill may mean to the patient not to exist, in which case the denial of illness results in the feeling of existing.

This point of view has been criticized first in terms of the emphasis placed on motivational factors and secondly on the validity of denial as the unifying motivational factor (12, 13). In regard to the first point, there appears to be too great a tendency to interpret the patient's expression of his felt reactions rather than to accept them at face value as reflecting altered capacity for dealing with sensory input or disturbances in sensory input. The second objection raises two points: first, the validity of any unitary theory of motivation, and second, the important point overlooked that the occurrence of brain damage not only alters the language in which motivational factors are expressed, but also the nature of the motivation itself.

The holistic approach of Weinstein and Kahn, though based in part on the work of Kurt Goldstein (3), differs in several significant respects from the latter. Goldstein in a recent contribution (14) has made some of these differences more explicit.

From the organismic point of view symptoms are regarded as performances of the sick individual and are only in part explainable on the basis of dysfunction of limited parts of the brain. "Symptoms are the consequences of the sick organism's struggle with the demands of the tasks confronting it. Symptoms are forms of behavior by which the individual tries, in spite of his defect, to come to terms in the best way with the outer and inner world" (14, p. 771). In his analysis of the symptomatology of the brain-damaged patient, Goldstein emphasizes the impairment in abstraction or the capacity to assume the "abstract attitude" and the concreteness of the responses shown in these patients (the concrete attitude). In the latter "we are given over passively and bound to the immediate experience of unique objects or situations. Our thinking and acting are determined by the immediate claims made by the particular aspect of the object or situation" (14, p. 773). The abstract attitude implies by contrast the ability to transcend the immediate demands of the environmental situation, to shift one's line of thought voluntarily, to make choices, to plan ahead and to think or perform symbolically and to account to oneself for one's actions and to be able to verbalize the account. Goldstein sums this up as follows:

"In brief the patients are changed with respect to the most characteristic properties of the human beings. They have lost initiative and the capacity to look forward to something and to make plans and decisions; they lack phantasy and imagination; their perceptions, thought and ideas are reduced; they have lost the capacity for real contact with others, and are therefore incapable of real friendship, love and social relations" (15, p. 255).

Another significant observation is the occurrence of the "catastrophic reaction" or state of severe anxiety occurring when the patient is unable to master the task at hand. The significant element is the failure and not the importance of the task. Failure at any task can place the patient in what Goldstein also refers to as a "disordered condition." The important element in precipitating the reaction is the impossibility at that moment of "self-realization." It is important to emphasize that these patients do not behave like people in a state of fear—"that is, they do not intentionally try to avoid situations from which anxiety may arise" (15, p. 257). They cannot do so because to do so pre-supposes the ability to adopt the abstract attitude. This limitation also accounts for the patient's unawareness of defect, such as hemiplegia or hemianopia, and of the difference between his state prior to the development of the symptoms and his present state.

There is, however, in addition to this subjective lack of aware-ness, an effective exclusion from awareness. This latter occurs particularly "when the degree of functional defect in performance is extreme. We can say that defects are shut out from the life of the organism when they would seriously impair any of its essential functions and when a defect can be compensated for by other activities, at least to the extent that self-realization is not essentially disturbed" (15, p. 258).

Viewed in this manner, anosognosia, or unawareness of defect, is a secondary effect—secondary to the patient's passive constric-tion of his total sphere of thought and activity to those areas in relation to which he can realize himself, e.g., function without frustration and disorder. "Since these disturbances are reactions which represent all that the individual is able to execute, he recognizes them as fulfillment of the task; in that way, these reactions fulfill this need to such a degree that no catastrophe occurs. Thus the protection appears as a passive effect of an active 'correct' procedure and could not be correctly termed denial, which refers to a more intentional activity, 'conscious' or 'unconscious' " (15, p. 259). Within the ensuing new organ-ization of behavior the disturbance is not as apparent. The patient has arrived at a new "preferred position" which compensates for the defect.

Goldstein differentiates the protective mechanisms of with-drawal and avoidance and unawareness of defect in the brain-damaged patient from the defense mechanisms of the neurotic by emphasizing their passive involuntary origin in contrast to the more actively and consciously contrived neurotic mechanisms. The protective mechanisms are simply new modes of preferred behavior.

Actually the differentiation between protective mechanisms and defensive mechanisms, mentioned in several of Goldstein's writings, is not quite convincing inasmuch as defense mechanisms are usually thought of as originating involuntarily and unconsciously. At one point Goldstein himself negates the distinction in the case of neurotic children. Here he feels they may be acquired in a passive way and hence in a way which is similar to organic patients. If this distinction is blurred, then the avoidance Goldstein speaks of takes on the character of a psychological mechanism operating to protect the individual from an unpleasant affect. It would perhaps be more consistent with Goldstein's own point of view to relate both the initial difficulties in awareness of defect and the subsequent difficulties to the limitations imposed by the impairment in abstract attitude alone, without the notion of a teleological factor embedded in the term "a protective mechanism" even if it is qualified by saying it is passively acquired.

The various manifestations of unawareness of illness (anosognosia) and unawareness of the affected part (imperception of the limb or asomatopagnosia) as they are encountered in the stroke population are illustrated in the following protocols.

In the first patient the denial phenomenon occurred as one among many responses indicating confusion and disorientation:

> *Case 58.*   76 year old white male. Right hemiparesis. *Diagnosis:* Probable intracerebral hemorrhage, left side.
>
> On admission the patient was found to be aphasic and disoriented. No history was available. Examination revealed a right hemiparesis with increased deep tendon reflexes on the right and bilateral Babinski and confirmatory signs. Cerebrospinal fluid was xanthrochromic. EEG revealed an abnormal focus on the left side anteriorly.
>
> When the patient was seen a week after admission he appeared to be in poor contact with his surroundings and was disoriented for time and space. Attention span was very limited and speech was difficult to follow because of a tendency to mutter and mumble in an inaudible fashion. He gave the date as the 23rd of June, 1909 (actually November 12, 1959). He was unable to name the hospital or estimate how long he had been there. When asked why he came, his response was, "I wanted to come in for medicine."

Q.   What is your main trouble?
A.   I want to get my concession going.
Q.   What is your main trouble?
A.   I forget.
Q.   Is anything wrong with any part of your body?
A.   No, not yet.

Concreteness of thought, disorientation and misnaming are evident in the responses of the next patient:

Case 59.   68 year old white female. Mixed aphasia. *Diagnosis:* Seizure disorder with post-ictal transient hemiparesis and speech disorder.

No history was available on admission. The patient has been a known epileptic for the past 8 years. Examination revealed a severe mixed aphasia, dyslexia, and dysgraphia. Spontaneous speech was mostly jargon. Neurological examination revealed a right extensor plantar response and absent right abdominal reflexes. Cerebrospinal fluid was clear. The following exchange occurred in an interview three days after admission:

Q.   Where are you now?
A.   I'm here now.   (Concrete response.)
Q.   Where are you now?
A.   In the Saratoga Hotel.   I'm not far from my own home.
(Misnaming and disorientation.)
Q.   Where is your home?
A.   I live on Long Island.
Q.   What kind of a place is this?
A.   It's a sort of hotel.   Not a hotel exactly.   Not a classy hotel.   Not a real hotel.   (Paraphasic response.)

In the next patient, in addition to disorientation and concreteness of thought, there is a fluctuating pattern of denial of defect, personification of the affected limb and spatial reduplication:

Case 60.   73 year old white female. Left hemiplegia. *Diagnosis:* Thrombosis or embolism, right middle cerebral artery.

Onset of weakness of left side one week prior to admission. On admission the patient was drowsy and had no spontaneous speech. When stimulated, however, she could name objects presented to her. There was conjugate deviation of the eyes to the right and a left homonymous hemianopia. There was a hemisensory impairment in addition to the motor loss on the left side. There was a left plantar extensor response. When she was first asked the question "Have you any weakness in your left arm and leg?" her response was "No." When shown her left arm, she said it was hers and that it was paralyzed.

One week later the patient was more responsive. Disorientation for time and space was noted:

Q. What happened to you?
A. My stomach. (Patient does not spontaneously refer to the paralyzed side. Implicit denial.)
Q. What happened to you?
A. I got a kick in the pants. I'm 73 years old. My stomach is bad and I had a heart attack. I must have gotten a kick in the pants.
Q. Who did it?
A. The world.
Q. What hospital is this?
A. Norwalk Hospital.
Q. Where is it?
A. Norwalk, Connecticut.
Q. Where do you live?
A. New York City.
Q. How did you get here?
A. By car, a 1937 Plymouth. (Concrete response.)
Q. What happened to your arm?
A. It's queer.
Q. In what way?
A. It's out of commission. They say it's a stroke.
Q. What do you think happened?
A. I wouldn't be surprised.
Q. Is there anything wrong with your leg?
A. Nothing. (Initial denial response.)
Q. Move your leg. (The patient then moved her left leg, using her right arm.)
Q. Is there something wrong with your leg?
A. It's queer.
Q. Where were you born?
A. Brooklyn.
Q. What does your husband do?

A. He's a stage manager.

Q. Do you have any children?

A. No.

Q. How come you never had any?

A. I was never pregnant. (Concrete response.)

Q. What kind of work did you do?

A. I'm an actress. I worked until last year. (Confabulated response. Patient has not worked in many years.)

A week later the patient appeared brighter and more alert. She spoke with mingled affection and derision of her paralyzed arm and leg, often referring to them in the third person. She commented spontaneously: "I'd love to do something about this old leg of mine. It's kind of a stinker." On another occasion, as the examiner approached, she remarked, addressing her arm: "Get up, silly, come on, get up. Don't make a fool of me. Can you stay up? Don't make an exhibition of me. My morale is low because I'm in incessant pain. I'm looking forward to a long day's journey into another night. I can't move my left hand independently. It's very unpleasant—a very unpleasant sort of thing. Stop that nonsense! (Again talking to her hand.)

Q. Why are you talking to your hand?

A. So it should understand it belongs to me. You talk to your car when you want it to go.

Q. What does your arm feel like?

A. I don't feel it at all. It's unpleasant.

Q. What hospital is this?

A. It should be the Hollywood Hospital, in Norwalk, Conn. (The hospital is given a more euphemistic name and placed closer to her home.)

Q. What's today's date?

A. I don't know.

Q. What month?

A. Maybe July—the 4th of July, a Protestant holiday, my birthday. (Actually June 5, 1958.)

Q. What year?

A. 1958.

Q. When were you born?

A. 1891, July 12th.

Q. Where do you live?

A. At the moment in Norwalk, Conn.

Q. Why are you in the hospital?

A. I haven't the slightest idea. Somebody said it was a heart attack. Others called it a stroke. That's a terrible word. It's rather exaggerated. It has a menacing sound. Is there a Hollywood Hospital in New York? It could be on West Fourth Ave.

Q. Did you ever hear of Bellevue Hospital?

A. Yes, but I never knew it was in Norwalk. (Spatial reduplication.)

Q. Where is Bellevue Hospital?

A. In New York City. Twentieth Street and First Avenue, New York. The greatest city in the world. I never thought Bellevue had any connection to Norwalk.

Explicit denial of disability and of the affected part itself are noted in the next patient:

Case 61. 73 year old white female. Left hemiplegia. *Diagnosis:* Thrombosis, left middle cerebral-internal carotid system. Onset with sudden loss of consciousness. Neurological findings included a left homonymous hemianopia, left central facial weakness, left flaccid hemiplegia with severe hemisensory deficit, deep reflexes more active on the left side, left Hoffman sign, and bilateral extensor plantar responses. She was oriented for person and place and approximately oriented for time. When questioned initially there was explicit denial of illness:

Q. Why are you here?

A. I don't know. I had a fall two years ago.

Q. What is wrong with you?

A. I don't know. I just slipped and fell. Help me up and out of here.

Q. Is there anything wrong with you?

A. My back and head hurt.

Q. Anything else?

A. Not a thing.

Q. Any weakness?

A. Not a bit. I'm weak for something to eat or drink.

Q. Hold up your right hand. (Patient does so.)

Q. Hold up your left hand.

A. I'll get it in a minute. (Patient does nothing.)

Q. Hold your left hand up.

A. You never have to use the left hand like the right. Nobody does. (Rationalization.)

Q.   But can you move the left hand?

A.   It's not paralyzed.   (Explicit denial of disability.)

Q.   Why are you not moving it?

A.   That's the arm I fell on.

Q.   I believe your left arm and leg are paralyzed.

A.   No, doctor.   I would tell you if I felt it.

Soon after admission a breast carcinoma was discovered. She was treated with irradiated gold. Her mental status showed some improvement during the next three months. At the end of that time the following interesting exchange took place. The patient was interviewed at the bedside. Her left hand was covered by the bedclothes.

Q.   What is your main trouble?

A.   My left side.   I can't use it.   My arm has no hand. (Denial of the affected part.)

Q.   What happened to your hand?

A.   A stroke.

Q.   Where is it?

A.   I never saw it.

Q.   There it is.   (The examiner takes the left hand from under the cover.)   What is that?

A.   That's what's on there.   I don't call it a hand because it holds nothing.

Q.   What do you call it?

A.   I guess I must have called it an arm.   (Patient keeps looking to the right side.)

Q.   Is it your arm?

A.   Yes, because the pain comes and lets me know it's mine.

Q.   What is today's date?

A.   I wouldn't know.

Q.   What year is it?

A.   1959.   (The date was November 5, 1959.)

Q.   What is your address?

A.   1 - - West 7 - - Street. This house here is my address. (Concreteness.)

Q.   How far is your house from here?   (Actually about 5 miles.)

A.   I only have to go downstairs and ring the bell. (Spatial disorientation.)

Q.   What kind of a place is this?

A.   A hospital.

Q. How do you know it is a hospital?
A. I'm in it and sick. You ask such silly questions. I know
it's a hospital now—I know it well.

In the next patient ownership of the limb was denied and
bizarre rationalizations were offered with an otherwise apparently
clear sensorium. Impairment of abstract attitude was readily
demonstrable.

> *Case 62.* 74 year old white male. Left hemiparesis. *Diag-
> nosis:* Thrombosis, right internal carotid—middle cerebral
> system.
>
> Patient is a known alcoholic and has had many previous
> admissions to the hospital. Earlier diagnoses included hyper-
> tensive cardiovascular disease, arteriosclerotic heart disease and
> cirrhosis. Auricular fibrillation was noted two years ago. Patient
> appeared acutely ill on admission (May 9, 1960) and was unable
> to give a coherent story. Cerebro-spinal fluid was clear and
> under normal pressure. Patient was drowsy but could be awak-
> ened. Neurological findings included pinpoint, unreactive
> pupils, a left homonymous hemianopia, paralysis of the left
> seventh nerve, diplopia on left lateral gaze, and a left hemi-
> paresis and left lower facial. The tongue deviated to the right.
> There was impairment of pinprick on the left. Deep reflexes
> were slightly increased on the left. There was a right extensor
> plantar reflex and the abdominals were absent on the left.
>
> The first psychiatric interview was held on June 1, 1960.
> The patient appeared to be well oriented for time, place, and
> person. He was not questioned about his left hand at this time.
> The only clue to mental deficit occurred when he attempted
> to give an account of his present illness. He was somewhat
> vague, spoke about his drinking, and had no insight into what
> had really happened.
>
> The second interview took place on June 8, 1960:
> Q. What is your main trouble?
> A. All my muscles hurt me. I was up all day—it was pretty
> windy. It's just like needles going all through my body.
> (The patient was lying in bed. His left hand was protruding
> from under a blanket. He spontaneously remarked:)
> "When I got put in bed this arm was sticking out. I told
> the nurses and doctors. They think it's my arm, but it's not.
> That's been sticking out like this ever since I was put in here."

Q. Whose hand is it?

A. I wouldn't know. It was here when they put me in bed. I always had an idea I was laying on top of a corpse because this hand was laying out there motionless.

Q. Where is your left hand?

A. Right here. (Patient began looking and groping. He touched his left arm.) I don't know. That's not mine. It's always hidden behind this. (Left arm.) That's been a mystery ever since I came in. If I touch it I can feel it, but it's not connected with my upper shoulder.

Q. Where are you now?

A. Bellevue Hospital.

Q. What kind of a place is this?

A. I called it Hotel Bellevue the other day. Everybody was eating in the dining room. (Paraphasic misnaming.)

Q. What kind of place do you think it is now?

A. Hospital.

Q. Are you sure?

A. Positive.

Q. How do you know?

A. There are doctors and nurses. You find them in a hospital or in saloons.

Q. Why did you come to this place?

A. I came home Sunday. I left the keys inside. I had a couple of drinks. I broke the door down. I sat on a chair. I fell off the chair and hit the floor. My landlord came. He picked me up and called a cop.

Q. What did you think was happening?

A. I really didn't know.

Q. Were you sick?

A. I wasn't sick.

Q. Are you sick now?

A. I don't know whether I'm sick or not. Every bone in my body hurts me.

The patient estimated his hospital stay as two weeks. (It was actually four weeks.) He was able to do simple problems and answered questions concerning current events appropriately.

Q. Who would have left an arm there?

A. I can't understand unless someone was operated on and they threw it right in with him. I once thought it was a urine bottle.

Q.   Do you know whose hand it was?

A.   How could I know? It was there when I got here.

Q.   Whose hand does it look like?

A.   I don't know.

Q.   Does it seem strange to you?

A.   You're telling me! It's the strangest thing I ever saw. I asked the doctors and nurses. Nobody ever said a thing about it. We're so close to the ferry that brings bodies over to Potter's Field maybe they threw one out sometime.

Q.   Do you have any other ideas about it?

A.   Well, the morgue is not far from here. I've never been there.

Q.   What is the difference between these two hands?

A.   That's (the left hand) not attached to my body.

Q.   What kind of work do you do?

A.   Painting. It's a funny thing—I did all those law offices. I worked right here at 8 - - Eighth Avenue.

Q.   That's not the address of this building.

A.   Of course it is.

Q.   How could it be on Eighth Avenue and be Bellevue Hospital at the same time?

A.   I understand it's a branch office. (Spatial reduplication.)

Q.   Where is your left hand?

A.   I don't know. I can't find it. Sometimes I think I'm laying on top of it. Sometimes I think there's another guy underneath.

At an interview on June 15th, the patient seemed to be even more uncertain as to whether or not the hand belonged to him. He registered annoyance at the examiner's persistent questioning:

Q.   Whose arm could it be?

A.   I don't know. You asked me that a hundred and sixty times. I don't know. It was in my bed. I couldn't use it. So it couldn't be mine. I woke up in the morning and it was there. Now I'm laying right on top of it.

Difficulty in abstraction was apparent in the handling of the following proverbs.

A stitch in time saves nine: "A stitch in time saves nine. They all come together."

People in glass houses shouldn't throw stones: "Because a stone is liable to be thrown back at them and break the house."

A rolling stone gathers no moss: "Because the moss doesn't get a chance."

Sensory examination repeated on June 16th revealed the following findings: There was a left hemisensory defect for pinprick. Vibration was perceived correctly at the shoulder, less well at the elbow, and not at the fingers. Position sense was lost at the fingers, wrist, and elbow. In the interview of that date the following exchange took place:

Q. How does your left arm feel?

A. As if it's hooked up here to the shoulder.

Q. Why do you think it's your arm now?

A. I'm not sure yet. It has to be proven to me.

Q. Whose arm is this? (The left arm is raised by the examiner.)

A. I don't know. It's too large to be mine. (There is dorsal edema of the hand.) And it's a right hand, not a left.

Q. Where is yours?

A. I feel it's underneath here. (Pointing to left forearm.) I never can reach it. I miss it. I always feel I have something in it.

Q. Did you ever see me before?

A. I think I did.

Q. What kind of work do I do?

A. You ask me a lot of questions.

Q. What kind of work?

A. Investigator.

Q. What kind of investigator?

A. To see if my brain still functions. In other words, if I'm ready for the nut house or the insane asylum.

Toward the end of June there was a clearer and more certain identification both of the arm and the existence of a paralysis. At the same time the patient's mood was one of growing irritability and annoyance mainly expressed toward the ward personnel. On June 28th, the following exchange took place:

Q. How does your arm feel?

A. It's limp-like. I can move the leg a little. The arm I can't do a damn thing with.

Q. Did you have a stroke?

A. It must be. I can't figure it out. I didn't have anything wrong with me before that happened.

Q. Do you ever still have the feeling that the arm is not yours?

A. I don't know. I can feel it up to the shoulder, but next to the shoulder there's no feeling. It's still a mystery to me. They must have sewn it onto me.

In the next patient a dysarthria was present, but was persistently denied. Although there were some inaccuracies in memory and orientation, neither the mental deficit nor the neurological findings were severe enough to account for the persistent anosognosia for her altered speech on the basis of either perceptual disturbances or impairment of abstract attitude. Furthermore, when she was actively challenged on this point she became defensive and hostile. Because of this it was felt that the continued unawareness of her speech impediment was primarily related to motivational factors rather than to the brain damage itself.

Case 63. 53 year old white female. Dysarthria. Mild right hemiparesis. *Diagnosis:* Thrombosis, basilar artery.

Onset occurred three days prior to admission, with a tendency to fall to the right. On admission she appeared alert and co-operative. Neurological findings: left lid drop, limitation of the right lateral gaze, right central facial weakness, deviation of tongue slightly to the right, mild but definite dysarthria, right hemiparesis, deep reflexes slightly increased on the right, abdominal reflexes absent, equivocal right Babinski, slight dysdiadokinesis left hand, slight terminal ataxia on finger to nose test on left. Cerebrospinal fluid was clear and under normal pressure.

The patient was born and raised in the South. She completed two years of college and then left to study singing in New England first, and then in Italy. She began her career as an opera singer at the age of 22. She continued to work professionally as an opera singer until ten years ago, when she had to retire because of illness (arthritis). She has been married for 28 years and has a daughter of 27. Her main interests center about music. When questioned about her illness she replied: "I tend to push it away. I never went to a doctor in my life."

The psychiatric interview was held 13 days after admission. The patient was able to give a coherent account both of the onset of her illness and the significant events in her own past history:

"I was home. I just happened to fall to the right. The maid

was there. She got the elevator man and put me back to bed. I lay down until my husband came."

Q. What did you think was happening to you?

A. I didn't know.

Q. Did you have any idea?

A. None, but my husband thought it was a stroke.

At one point in the interview, when her speech was particularly indistinct and difficult to understand, this fact was mentioned to the patient. She became flustered and annoyed, and in a somewhat indignant tone insisted that her speech was no different than it had ever been. Continued questioning provoked further irritation and annoyance.

When seen the following day she was asked to read a paragraph selected at random from a magazine. The dysarthria was particularly noticeable in the context of the reading material with which she was not familiar. She became impatient with the task and accounted for the very obvious difficulty she was having on the basis of poor vision and inability to see the print on the page. In actuality, the patient had no trouble at a visual level, but simply could not enunciate the words clearly when asked to read aloud.

Compare the following patient's response to that of the preceding one when challenged on their own statements concerning their defect.

Case 64.   74 year old white female. Left hemiparesis. *Diagnosis:* Thrombosis, right middle cerebral-internal carotid system.

Patient suffered a cerebrovascular accident while convalescing from a nephrectomy and splenectomy. She developed a left hemiparesis and became uncooperative, disoriented and resistive. Sensory examination was unsatisfactory. Pinprick and light touch could be appreciated in all areas. When seen ten days after the onset of the stroke, she appeared improved and was able to sit up in a wheelchair with restraints. She was responsive when questioned, but did not seem very aware of or interested in her surroundings:

Q. What do you feel is wrong today?

A. I'm no good.   I want to be out of this harness.

Q. What is wrong?

A. The spine is pressing.

Q. Anything else?

A. I bumped my head and it's sore.
Q. Any weakness?
A. No, no weakness.
Q. Are your left arm and leg O.K.?
A. They appear to be.
Q. Have you ever had any weakness in them?
A. Never noticed any.
Q. Show me your left hand.
A. Here it is. (Looks towards it.)
Q. Raise your arm.
A. (No response.)
Q. Raise your arm.
A. It takes some effort for me to do that.
Q. Why?
A. I don't know. I can't make the effort. The arm doesn't seem to be in me. I mean I can't do it. I would have to sit up more to do it.

The disorientation and clouding of consciousness gradually disappeared over a period of two months. The patient became aware that she had had a stroke and was now paralyzed. With this awareness a depressive and apathetic reaction set in. When asked to compare the way she was formerly with how she felt now, she replied: "I was free and easy, full of life. I'm a different person now altogether. My memory is gone. I'm not as fussy as I was. I don't care. Everything about myself that should be taken care of, like personal things, I forget. I don't care about taking care of myself. I'm just so down I can't get up."

Observations such as those described above and of other patients who exhibited denial phenomena led to certain general formulations:

(1) All of the patients in this category initially showed some evidence of diffuse brain dysfunction. In none did the phenomenon occur in the presence of a perfectly clear sensorium and without any impairment in abstract attitude.

(2) The anosognosic response has to be viewed as a dynamic process extending in time. The initial state of unawareness of either the deficit or the affected parts themselves occurs as a direct result of the impairment in abstract attitude in a situation

in which altered perceptual experiences are occurring.

(3) The motivational factors influencing the integration of the initial experience and the subsequent behaviorial manifestations differ from person to person. In some patients these initial reactions are exploited in the service of the need to deny illness. In others, however, one gathers the impression that they simply persist as sensory effects in an individual who is handicapped in his ability to grasp the newness of his experience, to bring it into line with other relevant associative data and to integrate the altered perceptual effect at an insightful level. The outside observer notes the paralyzed limb and visually perceives its attachment to the body of the patient. The patient experiences the paralyzed limb in its foreign-ness, strangeness and separateness from his body. He is unable to correct these impressions visually as he has not been able to experience them in their "new" significance. To do so would involve an abstract maneuver of which he is incapable. The initial response either endures unchanged or if general improvement occurs, it is gradually superseded by a more adequate awareness of his altered circumstances.

(4) The use of the term "denial" should be limited to those situations in which this specific motivational pattern clearly dominates the picture. The term "anosognosia" would thus have a different connotation and would apply to those situations of unawareness resulting from the combination of altered perceptual experience occurring at a time when, as a result of diffuse brain dysfunction and associated impairment of abstract attitude, there is an inability to conceptualize the new experience in new terms. The explanations offered by the patient, which appear to the outside observer as rationalizations, represent attempts to describe the felt reactions in concrete terms associated with past situations which in one or more ways resemble the felt reactions of the current situation.

CHAPTER X

THE POTENTIAL ANOSOGNOSIC RESPONSE

Transitory anosognosic and transitory personification responses appeared to have several common factors in their development. They were associated with sensory and motor deficits occurring in a setting of diffuse cerebral dysfunction. The fact that these responses may occur in a transitory fashion suggested that they may be more common than is generally believed to be the case, and may, perhaps, be frequently overlooked. As an outgrowth of our interest in differentiating between motivated denial responses and these initial anosognosic and personification reactions, we then concerned ourselves with the question of identifying elements of these latter two responses as they may appear in patients with no overt anosognosic or denial syndromes (12).

A series of interesting responses was obtained when patients who had residual motor deficits, but who did not show "denial" phenomena, were questioned about their subjective reactions to the hemiparesis or hemiplegia. The inquiry was divided into two parts. First an attempt was made to elicit the patient's subjective reactions to the affected part. Following this, a series of questions was asked to see whether or not certain specific effects had been noted by the patient if they had not been spontaneously reported. The questions asked were as follows:

Part I:

(1) At the time you became ill, tell me in detail the very first thing you noticed about your right/left arm/leg.

(2) Was there any other way in which your arm/leg was different from the other arm/leg?

(3) Did you notice anything else peculiar or strange about the arm/leg?

Part II:

(1) Did your arm/leg ever feel as if it/they were dead?

(2) Did your arm/leg ever feel as if it/they were not part of your body?

(3) Did it/they ever feel as if it/they did not belong to you?

(4) Did it/they ever feel as if it/they were someone else's arm/leg?

Sixty-seven such patients were given this questionnaire; 35 gave positive responses to one or more of the last three questions of Part II. Upon inquiry, they admitted to having transient feelings to the effect that the arm or leg felt separated from the body, as if it didn't belong to them or as if it belonged to someone else. Descriptions of this nature were termed *the potential anosognosic response* as they appeared to be the anlage or precursor of what, under conditions of greater brain damage and diffuse dysfunction, emerged clinically as either anosognosia or imperception of a bodily part. Positive responses to the first question of Part II alone were not considered significant. The effects described by these 35 patients occurred in a setting characterized by a clear sensorium and insight into the subjective nature of what they were experiencing. In many instances their responses often represented their first attempt to conceptualize the subjective impact of the sudden and unexpected motor loss. The more severely brain-damaged patient appears to objectify or concretize felt reactions which under conditions of less impairment are simply subjective accompaniments of a disease process.

Nine patients (Part I) spontaneously described effects that were similar to those elicited when affirmative replies were given in Part II.

In the first 34 patients who were given the questionnaire, 15 gave the potential anosognosic response and 19 did not. These two groups were compared with respect to neurological and electroencephalographic findings and no significant differences were noted.

Some of the characteristic affirmative responses were the following:

"It was just like the side didn't belong to me. It was like there was another person over there that I couldn't feel."

"It didn't feel like mine. It felt like a dead animal, I guess."

"When the pain comes that's when you know it's part of your body. Otherwise it doesn't feel like it's a part of you."

"It felt like I had no arm at all on this side."

"It didn't feel like mine. It felt like a piece of dead meat dragging on my neck."

It is important to emphasize that these patients were describing a transient perceptual experience occurring in the light of full consciousness. The uniformity of their responses, the directness with which they were presented, the absence of secondary elaboration and of any associated behavioral manifestations of denial suggest that these patients were simply involved in the effort to describe a form of sensory experience. In the absence of diffuse cerebral dysfunction, these effects are minimized and compensated for by other perceptual and cognitive data. These abnormal effects are crowded out by the weight of past experience and the remaining normal afferent input. Expressed in another way, the relevant motivational need of these patients was not to deny but to state to themselves with greater or lesser clarity the impact of a sudden and dramatically new form of experience.

We might sum up the sequence of events occurring in the wake of a stroke associated with a motor deficit in the following manner:

(1) Altered sensory and motor effects are experienced by the patient.

(2) These altered perceptual experiences form the basis for the potential anosognosic response.

(3) Whether or not these perceptual experiences are corrected, e.g., integrated at an insightful level, depends on two factors:

    (a) Does the patient have the capacity to make such a correction?

    (b) Does the motivation exist to make the correction?

(4) The capacity in turn is a function of two related factors:

    (a) Has any alteration occurred in the general capacity, e.g., any impairment of abstract attitude?

    (b) How severe is the motor and sensory loss?

(5) The motivation likewise is dependent upon two sets of interrelated factors:

(a)   The premorbid personality.

(b)   The current life situation.

(6)   The interplay of capacity and motivation determines the final resultant:

(a)   Patients may integrate the experience at a realistic level.

(b)   Patients may submit in a passive and resigned manner.

(c)   Patients may struggle to deny the fact and implications of illness.

(d)   Patients may be unable to cope with the illness in any of the above three ways because of impairment of abstract attitude and their consequent inability to relate themselves to the motor deficit as a new and significant event in their lives (Cf. accompanying chart).

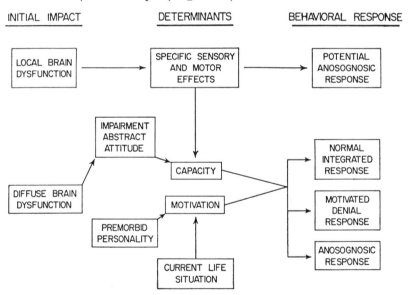

What Critchley (6) refers to as the "curiously detached attitude of the hemiplegic" or what emerges more explicitly as "denial" may come about as a result of very different mechanisms. A patient may be unaware of a deficit such as hemiplegia because it is expedient for him in a psychological sense to relate to the deficit in this manner. On the other hand, the unawareness may signify an actual inability to become aware owing to impairment in abstract function.

CHAPTER XI

CONCLUSION

Over two decades have elapsed since the author was an interne and had under his care a number of elderly patients with cerebrovascular accidents. As I recall, these patients were generally regarded by the house staff as the least interesting both from the standpoint of diagnosis and of treatment. They seemed indescribably old and beyond the pale of any effective therapeutic regime. Communication was difficult. Nursing care was difficult. Disposition was difficult and, most important of all, finding the time to spend with these patients was difficult. Perhaps more subtle factors entered into the aversive reaction, factors having to do with the young physician's tendency to turn away from illnesses associated in his mind with final and inexorable degenerative processes.

Returning to an intensive study of this patient population after a lapse of time is a chastening experience. If the preceding pages have in any way intimated how much there is to learn about these patients, about the origin of their symptoms, about their needs—physical, psychological, and social—then they will have achieved their purpose.

To the physician stroke patients pose a series of unique challenges at many different levels, challenges which all too often go unrecognized and therefore unheeded.

They are challenging from a diagnostic point of view, although this aspect of the problem has not been germane to the present study. New concepts of vascular insufficiency, greater awareness of prodromal symptoms, increased recognition of basilar artery and internal carotid artery disease, the increased need for differentiating thrombosis from hemorrhage in view of the possibility of anticoagulation, have all added new dimensions to the problems of diagnosis, medical management and possible surgical intervention.

As pointed out in the last two chapters, these patients are challenging from the standpoint of the interplay of neurological and psychological features in shaping the behavioral sequelae. The still controversial interpretation of anosognosia is a case in point. Of particular concern to the psychiatrist is the very great need which exists in almost every patient for support, encouragement, guidance and, in some instances, more definitive intensive psychotherapy. It very soon became apparent in the course of the initial interviews with these patients that a number of indications existed for psychiatric help.

(1) The routine history taking on admission by members of the house staff for diagnostic purposes does not tap the reactive and often turbulent emotional state accompanying the initial phase of a stroke. It was very easy to establish rapport with these patients, and in fact most of them welcomed the show of interest and concern in their own feelings about what had happened to them. This type of exchange was the initial bridge in establishing a rapport that was important later in helping the patient face problems arising in the rehabilitation process and the anxieties associated with the vicissitudes of effecting a proper disposition.

(2) The psychiatrist can often be of help to the various members of the rehabilitation team in interpreting the reactions of the patient that obstruct or impede the rehabilitation process. Value judgments concerning the patient's motivations are sometimes premature or inappropriate in situations where the difficulties encountered may be reflections of subtle personality changes resulting from the brain damage. As Goldstein has emphasized, these patients are very adept at covering up mental deficits and giving the appearance of greater intactness than actually exists. Allowance has to be made for distractibility, limited attention span, or the tendency to perseverate in a task. The patient may be able to make progress when the task is simplified or when only one task is given at a time. The importance of avoiding failure and precipitating a catastrophic reaction must always be borne in mind.

(3)   Masked depressions and other reactive features may limit the cooperation of the patient. They can be brought to light and treated both by supportive psychotherapy and the judicious use of anti-depressants, stimulants and other drugs.

(4)   When disposition other than return to the home becomes necessary, severe reactions can be anticipated and handled. The patient's misconceptions concerning the implications of placement and his unawareness of what may be potentially positive in the situation can be brought into focus. When the patient's needs are more accurately known, a more appropriate and congenial placement may be effected.

(5)   Often in the case of patients returning home a meaningful psychotherapeutic relationship can offset the feelings of inadequacy, uselessness, and self-derogation and help the patient move in the direction both of a realistic evaluation of work possibilities as well as exploration of the remaining potential for new areas of accomplishment.

(6)   The psychiatrist familiar with the patient and his home milieu can often be of great help to the individual members of the patient's family in helping them understand and manage some of the disturbing manifestations of the patient, such as apathy, excessive dependency, attitudes of blame and irritability.

(7)   There are, of course, a number of instances in which frank psychiatric sequelae occur which require evaluation and disposition. Frequently these go unrecognized for too long a time and take a great toll of both the patient and his family.

(8)   At a social level, the psychiatrist as a member of the medical team caring for these patients also bears the responsibility for working toward the establishment of more adequate community resources for these patients, particularly following discharge from the hospital. The rehabilitation process should not end with nursing home placement. There is a great need for sheltered workshop programs, particularly for the younger age group.

A final challenge posed by these patients relates to the many avenues for future research to be explored until a deeper understanding is achieved of the actual impact and effect of a stroke upon the patient. There are many aspects of the symptomatology of which we know very little. Such is the case with the very important and frequent finding of aphasia. There have been no large-scale studies from a psychiatric point of view of what happens in the lives of these patients. In terms of the symptom itself, there has been no real breakthrough in retraining procedures.

Another problem relates to the psychiatric classification and diagnoses in this age group. There is no consistent and reliable way of evaluating the premorbid personality of an individual who has lived seven, eight, nine, or even ten decades.

One question raised and still unanswered in our own studies is why some patients show the potential anosognosic response and others do not. The broader questions of the interplay of structural and motivational factors require considerably more investigation. Still unclear is the question whether or not parietal lobe pathology exerts any special influences in the reactions of unawareness, avoidance, and spatial inattention as suggested by recent animal studies (16).

In closing, I would like to quote a pertinent observation made by Stanley Cobb:

"This common neurological disorder [the stroke] is borne by some with courage and equanimity. Others are thrown into a deep depression. The variability of reaction is rarely a question of the type or location of the lesion, but an expression of the whole life experience of the person who gets the stroke" (17, p. 553).

I might add that the courage Cobb speaks of cannot be localized in the distribution of any particular cerebral artery, and when it appears it is quite indestructible.

BIBLIOGRAPHY

1. Lee, P. R., Groch, S., Untereker, J., Silson, J., Dacso, M. M., Feldman, D. J., Monahan, K., and Rusk, H. A.: An Evaluation of Rehabilitation of Patients with Hemiparesis or Hemiplegia due to Cerebral Vascular Disease, *Rehabilitation Monograph* XV, the Institute of Physical Medicine and Rehabilitation, New York University-Bellevue Medical Center, 1958.

2. A Classification and Outline of Cerebrovascular Diseases (A Report by an ad hoc Committee established by the Advisory Council for the National Institute of Neurological Diseases and Blindness, Public Health Service), *Neurology, 8:5*, 1-34, May, 1958.

3. Goldstein, K.: *The Organism,* American Book Company, New York, 1939.

4. Weinstein, E. A., and Kahn, R. L.: *Denial of Illness,* Thomas, Springfield, 1955.

5. Babinski, J.: Contribution à l'Etude des Troubles Mentaux dans l'Hémiplégie Organique Cérébrale (Anosognosie), *Rev. Neurol.,* 27:845-847, 1914.

6. Critchley, M.: Personification of Paralyzed Limbs in Hemiplegics, *Brit. Med. J.,* 2, July 30, 1955, 284-291. (Cf. also Critchley, M., *The Parietal Lobes,* Edward Arnold, London, 1953.)

7. Head, H., and Holmes, G.: Sensory Disturbances from Cerebral Lesions, *Brain, 34:*102-254, 1911.

8. Pick, A.: Ueber Störungen der Orientierung am eigenen Körper, in Arbeiten aus der psychiatrischen. *Klin. Prag.,* Berlin, Karger, 1908.

9. Denny-Brown, D., Meyer, J. S., and Horenstein, S.: Significance of Perceptual Rivalry Resulting from Parietal Lesion, *Brain, 75:*433-471, 1952.

10. . . . ., and Banker, B.: Amorphosynthesis from Left Parietal Lesion, *Arch. Neurol. & Psychiat., 71*:302-313, 1954.

11. Weinstein, E. A., and Kahn, R. L.: Symbolic Reorganization in Brain Injuries, in *American Handbook of Psychiatry* (S. Arieti, Ed.), Basic Books, Inc., New York, 1959.

12. Ullman, M., Ashenhurst, E. M., Hurwitz, L. J., and Gruen, A.: Motivational and Structural Factors in the Denial of Hemiplegia, *Arch. Neurol.,* Vol. 3, 306-318, Sept., 1960.

13. . . . ., and Gruen, A.: Behavioral Changes in Patients with Strokes, *Am. J. Psychiat,* Vol. 117, 1004-1009, May, 1961.

14. Goldstein, K.: Functional Disturbances in Brain Damage, in *American Handbook of Psychiatry* (S. Arieti, Ed.), Basic Books, Inc., New York, 1959.

15. . . . .: The Effect of Brain Damage on the Personality, *Psychiatry, 15*:245-260, 1952.

16. Welch, K., and Stuteville, P.: Experimental Production of Unilateral Neglect in Monkeys, *Brain, 81*:3, 341-347, 1958.

17. Cobb, S.: Personality as Affected by Lesions of the Brain, in *Personality and the Behavior Disorders* (J. McV. Hunt, Ed.), The Ronald Press Company, New York, 1944.

INDEX